Boosting Joy

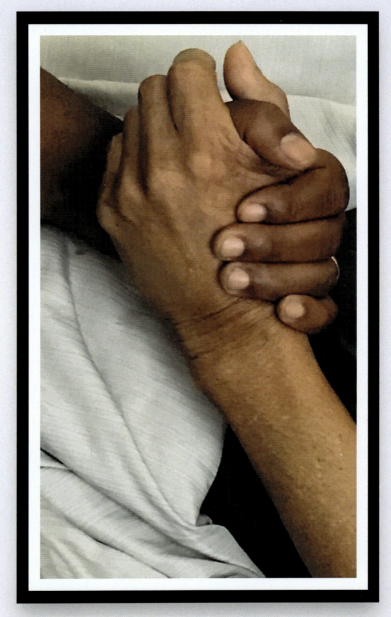

In the Grips of My Alzheimer's Caregiver Journey

Eunice L. Sykes

To order additional copies of this book, contact:
Xlibris
844-714-8691
www.Xlibris.com
Orders@Xlibris.com

Photos courtesy of Sykes family archives

ISBN: Softcover   978-1-6641-5993-8
        Hardcover   978-1-6641-5994-5
        EBook   978-1-6641-5992-1

Library of Congress Control Number: 2021903687

Print information available on the last page.

Rev. date: 08/16/2021

CONTENTS

ACKNOWLEDGEMENTS

This book would not be possible without the love and support of my family, extended family, church family, friends, and the many people whose paths I crossed during my Alzheimer's caregiver journey. I am amazed at the awesome work you do in the face of the enormous challenges you confront. May God continue to bless you. To the hospice organizations that were always there, thank you seems inadequate. Your work is invaluable. To my editing team, your deep dive and focus for this book is truly appreciated. I am forever grateful. For my beloved warrior husband Don, rest well.

This book is dedicated to loving caregivers everywhere.

PROLOGUE

I'm starting this journal in early 2011 as I'm about to embark on a journey that I know nothing about. This little diary is a sanity check for me, a reminder time and again that I must be the one to get there, even when I don't want to, even when I don't feel like it, even when I am overwhelmed. I haven't been this stressed in nearly 30 years. My earnest, fervent prayers are aloud yet almost silent, in hushed tones, rushed and on the run, but always necessary . . . some of them in Don's presence, with him adding his own petitions, especially in times of strife. So that God can calm us both down.

This journal entry and other passages in italics throughout this book were lifted directly from my in-the-moment notes and demonstrate where Don and I were on this journey. The book's format didn't come to me until fall in 2014, when I found myself praying constantly for guidance for a situation I had never encountered.

When I completed *Mashed Potatoes in My Salad: An Alzheimer's Caregiver Memoir*, the main character, Ramel, had met a man who seemingly complimented her, yet her future was left uncertain because of her loved one's Alzheimer's diagnosis. She was happy, restored, and on her way to living her best life *better*. This ending was full of wonder and hope, a hope that resonated with me personally, for the best outcome happened—Ramel and Mark are happily married and play plenty of golf between Georgia and Florida.

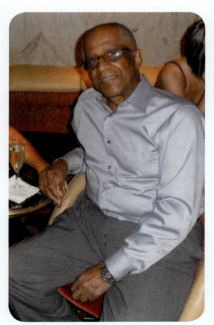

As for my own personal experience in "dementia-land," as I came to call it, my recordings were like those above: raw, detailed, and devastatingly personal anecdotes, feeling agonizing despair over what I was—no, *we* were—facing. I actually debated over and over whether to write this book. Alzheimer's disease or any type of dementia is a tough topic to talk about, let alone write about. With a timeframe unknown, I suspected the journey was going to be a rough ride, and I needed to fasten my seat belt. I came to realize that it was a blessing that my beloved soul mate, Don, the best husband I've ever had, eventually would not remember all of it like I would. Here he is before his diagnosis.

In many communities, folks do not speak openly about dementia. Having a stark and honest discussion rarely takes place. My exposure to dementia came when I was contracted years earlier to write someone else's story. Thus, I had to research and learn about it to write about it. To be honest, I didn't even know how to spell it. *Dimentia* was how I had written it before quickly learning of my mistake. As I read and absorbed what was to come, I came to understand there were many different forms of dementia. I also learned many startling facts from various resources, primarily the Alzheimer's Association. This organization provides vital care and support to those families facing the disease and supports critical research. The local chapter became my lifeline.

Hope was distant for me; I didn't know what to hope *for*. After all, the definition of *hope* reads that it is "the expectation that something good is going to happen at any moment." The world of Alzheimer's is like being at an amusement park. The journey includes gut-wrenching rides that fluctuate between merry-go-round moments to roller-coaster episodes, with spinning-top heights of dizziness and finally being knocked out breathlessly, an experience akin to the bottom dropping out of that speeding cylinder ride. Dementia of the Alzheimer's type is also like a freight train headed toward a deadly collision. The question is when.

One of my many prayers and scriptures in those many moments when I was absolutely inundated was Psalms 61:1–2, which reads, "When my heart is overwhelmed, lead me to the rock that is higher than I." Another was simply "Hear me Lord," taken from 2 Samuel 15. When my primal, most painful cries surfaced, "I Surrender All," a song from my youth, came to mind because I indeed have a rock in my Lord. Yes, it was something bigger than I that got me through this season, even when I felt I had nothing left, for I was sure that my "anchor holds and grips the solid rock."

Since my research indicated that an Alzheimer's diagnosis is a terminal diagnosis, how could I hope? What did hope even look like? This notion of hope was a constant, disappointing, and tough issue for me for over eight years as we battled the monster that would eventually take Don. We were both deeply spiritual people, and relying on our faith was like having an extra pair of hands. For that, I was grateful because our spirituality and humor would serve us well in the days and years to come. We owed it to ourselves to be as happy as we could be, whatever the circumstances.

I discovered that love and hope survive in helping others navigate their illness and their grief journey, both while loved ones are still walking the path and while they are at the moment of transition. This is not a journey of hope, but then maybe it could be. With such a profound loss emerging before your eyes, many hugs and much love, peace, turmoil, and laughter become constant companions, sometimes all at the same time. It is up to us to find the joyful moments and cling to them. It is up to us to discover hope in increments.

Don and I had such a beautiful relationship for twenty-six awesome years. They were full of fun, friendship, travel, worship, and golf. Don was a retired GE engineer for nearly twenty of those years; I was retired the last eight. When I relocated several times because of job promotions, Don suggested I consider places where he could engage year-round in one of his favorite hobbies—golf. I did! So for over eight years, we moved to Houston, Texas, Union, Kentucky, and Atlanta, Georgia, with a brief stint in Pittsburgh, Pennsylvania.

Hope eventually came in the form of a network of people and resources for us. Aside from the Alzheimer's Association, we discovered resources like support groups, the Alzheimer's Foundation of America, other dementia/Alzheimer's caregivers, social media (Facebook) private groups, websites, local events and activities, the veterans administration (VA), and various books, including my earlier book, *Mashed Potatoes in my Salad: An Alzheimer's Caregiver Memoir*. I delighted to see from the broad dementia community a willingness to share, educate, inform, dispel myths, and help in assuring others that they were not alone.

Scriptures from the Holy Bible came to me, often in the middle of the night, that sustained me, bolstered me, kept me, guided me, and comforted me. I did not yet realize that God would use my struggle for good. Prayer was key for me, though I often did not know what to pray for—was it strength, peace, or courage? I certainly did not want to be tested. I sought the answer to the following question: is God good when the outcome is not going to be? I came to know that my gift as a writer would allow me to reach people with a nonjudgmental message that would help them and encourage and support them with guidance, ideas, and recommendations. I hope this book does that. Perhaps there is something between these lines that touches you, inspires you, motivates you, and puts you in a better place. I truly believe that is what God would have me do with this experience; that is my purpose.

So after a year of healing, restoration, recharging, and regrouping following Don's transition, I began organizing a multitude of cherished handwritten or typed details from the backs of envelopes, Post-its, tablets, spiral notebooks, legal pads, magazines, and old computers and even on my cell phone. As is my custom, the handwritten notes were in shorthand, a long-ago throwback to my days as a business teacher. Since my youth, I have always used writing as a tool to understand, to record, to clarify, and to put things into perspective. Writing has always been a catharsis for me in my lifetime. I would feel some sense of relief, of comfort, but I knew there would be something more from this beyond just recording my journal entries.

Do not be unwise but understand what the will of the Lord is.
— Ephesians 5:17

As I labored and struggled with what to do with all this firsthand, raw, and candid text, I started recording nightly in 2011. God kept nudging me in the middle of the night. I frequently stirred with thoughts on my mind. I did not know why; I just did. Perhaps it was to document the unbelievable, to remember that which I didn't want to later recall. Perhaps it was to record what was happening, to try to make some sense of it, "it" being this devastating dementia disease called Alzheimer's. Putting my hands to paper oddly gave me some kind of control; writing lifted some of the burden, clarified my thinking, and helped me get ready for what was to come. Please know that in this journey, there will always be a "What's next?"

Like with childbirth, I labored, had many fits and starts, and breathed deeply as I reread words from years ago, wrestling to get a good foothold on how and where to begin. After much prayer and further discussions with trusted colleagues, I began writing thoughts, prayers, and songs and recording episodes to help me cope, capture the moment, stay sane, decompress, and gain fortitude for what was to come.

At the same time, several other incidents occurred during my journey that suggested I fine-tune my purpose: people began referring me to others on similar journeys, others called to inquire about resources, and friends and neighbors sought my help on interacting with Don. I did a podcast interview. I also noticed over time that while attending and learning much about dementia and Alzheimer's through various workshops, conferences, and forums, seldom did I hear the voice of the unpaid, loving caregivers, a critical and absolutely necessary component to this journey. I wanted to hear the perspective of the person spending the most time offering care and support to their loved one.

"For I know the thoughts that I think toward you," says the Lord, "thoughts
of peace and not of evil, to give you a future and a hope."
— Jeremiah 29:11

I wanted to do something about the stigma that exists in many communities where people do not talk openly about dementia. I have lived two lives in the dementia world and have much to say. My earlier book discussed dementia from another person's point of view. This book is *my* story, with a goal to share fun strategies designed to boost your joy over and over, to improve communications, to ease frustration and confusion, to lessen behavioral challenges, and to provide ideas on being creative for living your best life *better* for the rest of your life. Often while in the grips of Alzheimer's, boosting your joy is the last thing on your mind. This book offers nuggets to prepare you to face Alzheimer's. It is filled with joyful pictures, poetry for the caregiver, vignettes, and other sensitivities I experienced and took note of so that I would not forget and so that others could benefit, so that others could respond to the question "Where is the joy in this journey?"

As I struggled with whether to convert my journal entries into a book to share with others, I thanked God in advance for his grace and mercy while I recalled the words of two mentors. Dr. Maya Angelou said, "There is no greater agony than bearing an untold story inside you." Then Dr. John Hope Franklin personally told me years ago regarding an earlier published book, "Just tell the story." Finally, I was reminded of an old African proverb: "Until the lion learns how to write, every story will glorify the hunter."

Thus, I have written the book I wanted to read eight years ago—one that spreads hope, joy, education, enlightenment, inspiration, and encouragement and one that also reduces the stigma that I found connected to this disease. This book is the voice of the unsung hero, the loving care partner—a voice often missing in Alzheimer's public forums. It is for those just starting out on this journey who have no clue yet what to expect. If one person is helped and feels empowered to take things one day at a time, then my role is complete. I am blessed to be part of helping other caregivers, especially those dealing with dementia and specifically Alzheimer's, for it is a disease that consumes everyone concerned. This book is straight from my heart, the heart of someone who has been there, survived, and is thriving.

CHAPTER 1
Definitions

Once I began my research, I found plenty of information on these topics. Though I am not a medical professional, I do want to get us all on the same page of this disease. I recommend you do your own research to further complement your knowledge.

Dementia is the loss of cognitive function (thinking, remembering, and reasoning) and behavioral abilities to the extent that they affect daily living and activities. It is a slow decline in memory thinking and reasoning skills and is a fatal disorder that results in a gradual degeneration and shrinkage or loss of brain cells. There are no clear risk factors or identifiable causes to explain dementia development.

Alzheimer's disease is the most common form of dementia—it is responsible for 60 to 80 percent of all cases—and is one of the most critical public health issues in America. It is the sixth leading cause of death in the United States (and the fourth leading cause of death in African Americans). Some sources, for example the Alzheimer's Foundation of America, cite Alzheimer's as the leading cause of death in African Americans. Alzheimer's disease affects the hippocampus area of the brain. Neither dementia nor Alzheimer's is a mental illness.

This disease has no known causes and cannot be prevented, cured, or even slowed. Women are at the epicenter of Alzheimer's; women get it more often and are the dominant caregivers (thirteen million women in total). Every sixty-five seconds, someone in the United States develops the disease. More than 5.2 million Americans have Alzheimer's. Fifteen million Americans are providing unpaid care for a loved one with Alzheimer's. Only 45 percent of Alzheimer's patients or their caregivers report being told of their diagnosis. By 2050, Alzheimer's and other dementias will cost over $1.1 trillion. As this book is being published during the Coronavirus pandemic, more data on the impact of this virus will likely be adverse and worsen these numbers.

One in three seniors die with Alzheimer's or another dementia. Doctors are reluctant to cite Alzheimer's as the cause of death on the death certificate. Instead, they cite one of the results of Alzheimer's, like heart failure. This very important fact has a rippling effect as research findings for Alzheimer's funding are distorted or underreported because of the death citation. These numbers support grim, dismal statistics that have been prominent over the past twenty years, yet important strides are being made to move Alzheimer's research forward. Unprecedented funding makes research, care, and support possible in ways never before imagined. I am thankful that my husband, Don, played a small role in this research.

Alzheimer's is characterized and distinguished from other dementias by the existence and buildup of plaques and tangles in the brain known as tau and beta amyloid proteins. A medical MRI, PET scan, or lumbar puncture confirms whether these proteins exist.

In summary, two important pieces of information clearly affect this dreadful disease. Doctors seemingly are reluctant to cite a diagnosis of Alzheimer's. Also, when loved ones die of this disease, medical professionals are reluctant to cite Alzheimer's as the cause of death.

The Alzheimer's Association classifies the stages of Alzheimer's as early (mild), middle (moderate), and late (severe). There are other categories defined by others in the field. For simplicity, in this book, I will use the early (mild), middle (moderate), and late (severe) classifications.

Mild cognitive impairment or MCI is often the initial diagnosis from medical professionals when a patient presents himself or herself with memory issues. It is a brain disorder involving noticeable memory and other mental functions that are greater than normal, age-related changes. Though not as significant as a dementia diagnosis, MCI is often a forerunner of dementia. There is a fifty–fifty chance of MCI developing into Alzheimer's. MCI's common signs are forgetting things more often, losing track of a conversation, not remembering scheduled appointments, getting confused or lost when out and about, and increased difficulty in decision making, planning, or following directions.

With MCI, there is little interference with daily life and a person's ability to participate in daily activities. Often these problems are caused by certain medications, vascular issues, fatigue, strokes, urinary tract infections (UTIs), thyroid imbalance, chemotherapy, depressed moods, anxiety, and stress. Not everyone who has MCI will develop dementia. Lifestyle changes and choices—like exercise, proper diet, rest, and social interaction—may lessen the chances of developing MCI.

MCI was Don's first diagnosis in early 2014.

CHAPTER 2
Pre-Diagnosis

Bub . . . bub . . . bub . . . bub . . . bub . . .
Not getting better . . .
Death is coming for me soon . . .

I awakened one morning not knowing that this would be the last time I would know him as I did. It started with the first line above, which turned him into not knowing how to initiate, participate in, or finish a conversation. There was no name to this initially, but MCI was on its way to claiming my loving, funny, strong hubby, turning him into someone I did not know, did not recognize, and did not feel comfortable around. Thus, my caregiver stress journey began.

Yes, I observed many "episodes" in our daily lives that were not quite right, but I dismissed them and moved on. Was I in denial? Absolutely! But there was something about those words. As vague as they sounded, they were clear. Don and I were having a conversation while I washed dishes at the kitchen sink.

From that vantage point, Don came out of the bedroom, fifteen feet away, and I heard this never-to-be-forgotten utterance: "Bub . . . bub . . . bub . . . bub . . . bub . . ."

The Alzheimer's Association (source: www.alz.org) lists these ten warning signs for dementia:

- Memory loss that disrupts daily life
- Challenges in planning and organizing
- Difficulty with familiar tasks
- Confusion with time, day, and place
- Trouble understanding visual images and spatial relationships
- New problems with speaking words or writing
- Misplacing things and not being able to find them
- Decreased judgment
- Withdrawal from social activities
- Changes in personality

Alzheimer's disease knows no boundaries; it is classless, raceless, ageless, and an equal-opportunity attacker.

While the diagnosis was months away, Don did show these early signs of dementia. He was such an unlikely candidate for any kind of dementia, let alone Alzheimer's. At age seventy-three, he was an active exerciser, walking and/or golfing daily. Before and after his diagnosis, doctors often marveled at his physical presence, saying he had the body of a fifty-year-old man. He did. If, as a popular statistic indicates, walking cuts the chance of Alzheimer's in half, Don did not get that break.

Whenever I did well, I wanted to do even better.

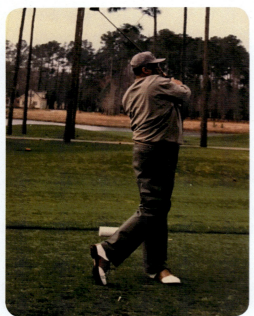

An electrical engineering graduate from the University of Kansas, he loved working at his computer, learning software and applying his knowledge to current projects. He also played his soprano saxophone, involved himself in various church ministries, took golf trips with his golf buddies, devoted time and money to charities, and was an avid card player who did his share of trash talking. Before retiring, he was an aeronautical engineer and computer professional. It was Don who had introduced me to the game of golf and thus into his life. We loved living in a golf course resort community, for golf was at the center of our lives. To know that the day would come when he would not know himself was mind-blowing to both of us. Meanwhile, we had to live our best lives *better*.

Along with sports of all sorts, Don loved animal shows. He enjoyed that slice of life as he struggled to come to terms with the grip that was tightening its hold on his being. With the children grown and on their own, we did everything together and separately. We had a robust spiritual and social life, traveled together and separately, entertained friends, became business partners, and thoroughly enjoyed each other. The uncertainty hovering over us still had no name at this point.

*I love my husband and want the best of the time we have left before I lose him entirely to this disease with no name yet. I want us to live our best lives **better** while we can.*

While noticing weight loss and more symptoms and a continual assault to his dignity over time, I discovered another scary statistic: once a person is diagnosed with dementia, they have actually been having symptoms for twenty years. The irony was that I had only known Don for twenty years, so I thought these personality quirks were cute. I had no other benchmarks. Don often laughed and chuckled his way through unfinished sentences. I accepted his reasonable excuses, humorous anecdotes, and common denial mechanisms. Along with his gradual short-term memory loss, there were signs of something else, something larger, looming. His language skills and recent behavioral changes indicated issues with higher levels of cognitive processing, prioritizing, and organizing.

Don struggled to concentrate; he became distracted by background noise, including someone else talking. He frequently left his yard work half-finished, and he scorched a ceramic storage container on top of the stove burner. His difficulty with assembling a new, shiny black corner unit desk for my office signaled something more. When I checked on him several times, he was in the same position: sitting in his chair, holding the instructions in his hand, with desk pieces strewn along the floor. He began hoarding toothpicks, toilet paper, and tissues and putting things in his pocket. He was always losing his glasses. I was puzzled and becoming more and more alarmed.

Dear God, bring peace into my home . . . let me not insist on correcting or being right or having the last word; let there be no more outbursts . . . in Your name.

He lost even more weight and was frequently confused with taking his pills. This began what I call the extremely difficult and pivotal pre-diagnosis stage. Don's frequent, unpredictable, and erratic behavior unnerved me. He was having these episodes daily and nightly. I had no clue about managing this still-yet-to-be-named monster that invaded our space and our place of peace.

Don turns on the water in the bathroom and walks away, headed to bed, where he rests . . . his spirit torn, his body ravaged, and occupied with his constant yet unnamed companion.

His bathroom habits and personal hygiene were beginning to suffer. His clothing choices and his difficulties in dressing himself were perplexing. Frequently, our conversations turned into outbursts that were surprisingly clipped and strained. Over time, as I got in my own way, he became increasingly aggravated and upset, often prompting the drop of the f-bomb.

He'd scream, "I feel like a f***ing child!"

I had never heard him curse. His memory problems, unclear thinking, and agitation caused our loving, intimate relationship to become tense in all aspects.

Love is not easily angered . . . must remember that. Love keeps no record of right or wrong . . . know that (Corinthians 13:4, paraphrased).

In the grips of what was happening, we both experienced moments of despair and a loss of who we were.

Lord, please help me to limit the rushed moments when Don is trying to think of his next word. To ask him if he wants my help. That's love. He utters, "Slow down," to himself when conversations don't come so easily. I also notice him taking the deep breaths I suggested as well. He's trying so very hard.

It still boosts my joy because throughout much of his illness, Don would intentionally pause, slow down, whisper to himself, and deeply breathe. I too would breathe (inhale, count to five, hold, count to five, exhale, count to seven) and pray, "Order my steps, Lord."

This was a time of discovery for the both of us. We had so many eye-opening and irritating moments. The episodes were not merely senior moments. What I had witnessed over time warned of a new reality: designing and building brick displays around our four trees that took an inordinate amount of time, purchasing duplicate yard tools, losing four cell phones and two gold rings, scrambling the TV remotes, walking with an impaired shuffle, forgetting to post and pay monthly bills, charging unusually large credit card amounts, and taking fewer walks through our lovely neighborhood. He misplaced things and could not track them down. He experienced personality and mood swings, and he avoided social activities. On the other hand, I had new tasks: closely monitoring the bills, the bank accounts, house maintenance, and his personal credit cards while my ignorance, insecurities, hopelessness, depression, and symptoms of stress crept into my being.

I woke up this morning prayerful and put a CD in the player: Roland Griffin, a gospel guitarist. He is bluesy with the songs I sang in my youth at St. Peters AME Church, like "Goin' Up Yonder" and

"He Looked Beyond My Faults." They resonate with a new, updated melody. Thank you, God, for being a mainstay in my life over these years and for keeping me at the cross.

I was frustrated, and Don was even more frustrated as he struggled with losing his pride and himself. He loved watching golf when he was not at the golf course. He could recite all the stats and lineups for most professional golf tournaments, a welcomed pastime and respite as he struggled to come to grips with his situation. My beautiful life was slowly slipping out of my reach, as evidenced by limited conversations, more time at home, stealing away to my closet for a moment of peace, remembering the feeling of what was, and acknowledging that it may never be again. My new outlets of release were screaming in the car before I got out of the driveway, crying while taking a shower, and shutting the door to a room for a moment of peace (until Don, who often "shadowed" me, appeared). I had few options to distribute this load I was under; I began my earnest search for better relief options immediately.

"Those who plan what is good find love and faithfulness" (Proverbs 14:20).

"I will never leave you nor forsake you . . . the lord is my helper; I will not fear" (Hebrews 13:5).

Though his memory is failing, Don is incredibly resourceful.

Despite all of this turmoil, Don's engineering mind, though befuddled, figured out how to keep aggressive birds from nesting (and messing!) on the column ledges on both sides of our front porch. He still found solutions for getting what needed to be "done, done," and preventing that bird poop from collecting all over the front porch was one of those moments of boosting joy. Years later, I am eternally grateful.

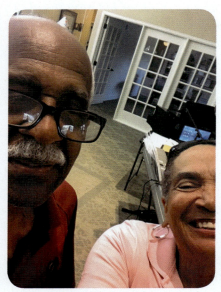

So I focused. *We* focused. We leaned on our spirituality and a generous dose of humor to keep some semblance of sanity along the way, as Don would often tease, "You're getting just like me." I responded with an often-used prayer: "Lord help us!" We both laughed hysterically at the thought. His petition was the same: "Lord help us."

*Trying to embrace this change in our relationship. It is not a welcomed guest. Rather, it is an intrusion, an adversary, a devastating disease with no cure. It is full of changes, changes for the worse . . . help me, Lord, to remember to put more fun and more life into our relationship. Help us to live our best lives **better**.*

Early on, I prayed for courage. I learned later not to pray for courage but instead to plead, "Lord, *be* my courage." I certainly did not want any more tests to build courage. Don was still somewhat independent at this time. He loved to go to the grocery store, located half a mile from our home. He would make a list, often misspelling simple words like *apples* ("appels"), his favorite fruit. Sometimes he got all the items on the list; other times, he did not. When I grocery-shop today,

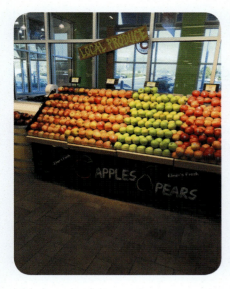

my joy surfaces when I approach the fruit section. I imagine Don meticulously picking the right apple.

He so wants to help out. "What can I do? How can I help?" Thank you, God, for Don in my life. Without him, I'm not sure where I'd be. I will see him, us, through this.

He would often return home after going out, and his black Nissan Altima would have new scrapes, dents, and scratches. One time the front right passenger mirror was dangling; another time, the back bumper was scratched. His decreased judgment when pulling into the garage far enough to clear the garage door was partially to blame. Prayer, always and again, became my constant companion. "Lord, I thank you for what didn't happen." Psalms 106:1 puts it this way: "O, give thanks, for his mercy endures forever."

When we went places together and he drove, I sat on the edge of my seat and gritted my teeth as he maneuvered close calls and unnecessarily slowed responses to traffic conditions. He would run red lights or stop fifty yards from the traffic light intersection. There were times when he took me to the store, dropped me off at the front door, and then parked and waited for me to shop. I loved having a chauffeur. When he saw me coming out of the store, he would approach and, with impaired judgement, run up on the sidewalk to make his turn alongside of me, damaging my front passenger tire area. Fear gripped me as his diminished driving skills clearly limited his errand runs. He sensed my anxieties and offered a tension-releasing shoulder or foot rub once we got home. I loved that!

Surely, I am wearing the weight of caregiving . . . I love it when you massage my shoulders or legs, Don.

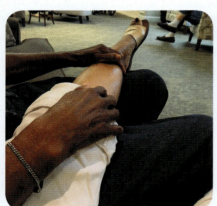

The episodes were never-ending, indicating problems far beyond simple memory loss. On one of my girlfriend golf trips, Don called to say that he was in a car accident and that the other person was at fault. His car was totaled. He indicated that a police officer brought him home after the car was towed. He never went to the emergency room. I wonder still whether that car accident exasperated his condition.

I am so disgusted with me. This disease is heartbreaking. As a care partner, I get so frustrated!

I watched, sadly, as Don took the ice bucket from the kitchen to the garage to wash his golf clubs, as he pulled a cotton turtleneck over a dress shirt, as he put on one pair of jeans, took them off, and put on another, and as he failed to recognize a four-pack tray of tomatoes on the kitchen counter when I suggested he have some with his dinner. He always had a glass of water and blessed his food, whether he was eating a tuna fish sandwich loaded with vegetables from Subway or Thanksgiving dinner.

In my ignorance, when I incorrectly attempted to correct him, he screamed, "You do your thing, I will do mine! You go your way, I'll go mine! Don't tell me what to do!"

I would scream back, "Pack your s**t!"

Okay . . . so this day, I didn't get it right. Yes, I came out of the gates wrong; my crown is skewed. It was just one of those days.

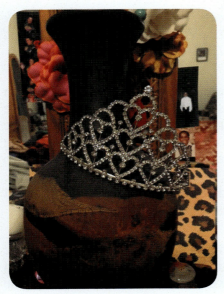

Neither of us meant those words. He had never raised his voice to me. I was often in tears.

After we both calmed down, I heard his cry as he paced back and forth, saying, "I try my best to do all I can to make things right."

I petitioned, "Lord, get me out of the way."

In the middle of the night, when I struggle to sleep, I notice near the window my laptop's amber light, blinking on and off like a beacon. I am comforted. When I want to pour my heart out, I use it to pour over these words.

Thank you, Father, for quiet, early morning hours when I can reflect and listen to your urgings, early morning meditations when all is still and I can hear your voice. Every time I feel the spirit, I am nourished. I am refreshed. I can go on . . . thank you sweet, sweet spirit. For when the spirit is moving in my heart, I will pray (paraphrased, another song from my youth).

Don often went to bed early; I believe he felt the onset of "sundowning," moody and irrational behavior symptoms during evening hours. Going to bed early was his response to minimizing it, but he was up and about most of the night, disrupting his sleep and mine. He wandered throughout the house most of the time, often passing the front door. At times when I asked him his date of birth, the current date, the day, and his name, he could not answer. He would shrug it off. I would look at him like "What the hell?" It was strange to me that a person could lose one part of their memory and yet remember things from a long time ago. Don spoke often of his nuclear family: his childhood, parents, brother, uncles, aunts, cousins, years growing up, even schoolmates. Clearly, I lacked understanding of what was happening and how this disease worked.

Thinking of a new future and a new you. You are slower. I need more patience. You're not thinking straight. I need more knowledge. You're not able to process. I must remember that. Need more direction. You're not holding your weight. I need more strength.

Another episode during this time that was significant was when we joined our church within a year of moving to Georgia from Pennsylvania. Membership during that year soared as over three hundred souls were brought to Christ, including Don and me. When the dynamic and anointed pastor asked us to share why we joined during a church district conference meeting, Don again exhibited signs of something wrong, even though he had notes. His speech was unclear; he hesitated and struggled to get words out. His short-term memory and focus were off once again. Somehow I was able to get us through this moment. I prayed for insight and clarity on what this madness was that had its grip on both of us. Both of us were deeply spiritual and continued participating in church ministries, like hosting the married couples ministry. Don continued his involvement in feeding the community and in the veterans' and communications ministries.

Philippians 4:6 tells us, "Be anxious for nothing . . . let your requests be known to God."

To encourage myself, I revisited a poem I wrote in 2000 called "Resilient":

Resilient is me—
A rubber ball,
An elastic band.
Stretch it.
Bounce it.
Bend it.
Extend it.
Snap it.
Slap it . . .
God, my soul to restore—
He is the one who makes me soar!
Then I come back again for more—
That's me.
Resilient is me.

Sometimes I believed that; sometimes I did not. Seemingly, the episodes ramped up when Don's only sibling, his brother, Abel Jr., died while living in an expensive, long-term care facility in Sacramento, California, after a long bout with another form of dementia (Parkinson's disease). We visited Abel several times over the years, and each time, his decline was more prominent than the previous visit.

At Abel's death, Don and I traveled to Kansas City, Kansas, his hometown, for the homegoing celebration. His parents were buried there. Don was to speak for the family, as he had done on similar previous occasions. Speaking of their loved ones, their nuclear family, used to come so easily to the brothers as they slid in and out of stories of their youth, their upbringing, with one tacking onto the other's words as they rhythmically rolled tales off the top of their heads. I was amazed at how these two sons intertwined their loving childhood stories of times with their wonderful father, Abel Sr. When his dear, devoted mother, Gladys, died, Don and Abel again celebrated her life with words, stories, and anecdotes from their youth. Before his dad's passing, I had never seen Don in a similar situation. I was both amazed and proud of him.

Things were different for Abel's service; Don fretted to put words about his only sibling onto paper. He'd never struggled like that before. In the days leading up to the service, time and again, he would write, ball up the paper, and toss it into the trash, thoroughly disgusted and disappointed. When we arrived in Kansas City, he still did not have any notes, yet at the service, Don was able to get through his comments with his dear nieces at his side. I had no clue what was going on. This was different.

Through it all, Don continued golfing but with added episodes, like leaving his clubs in the cart when he completed his round, leaving his trunk open during his round, or locking his keys in the trunk of his car. One of his golf buddies and I began coordinating these outings, getting him to the golf course, making sure that he had all his clubs, that he was registered, and that his golf rounds were pleasant.

When I asked how Don did one day, his friend honestly replied, "Okay but not like he used to."

Still, Don got his second hole in one while struggling with his favorite hobby. I'm not sure he realized what a joyful moment that was, hitting a once-in-a-lifetime shot! I certainly did.

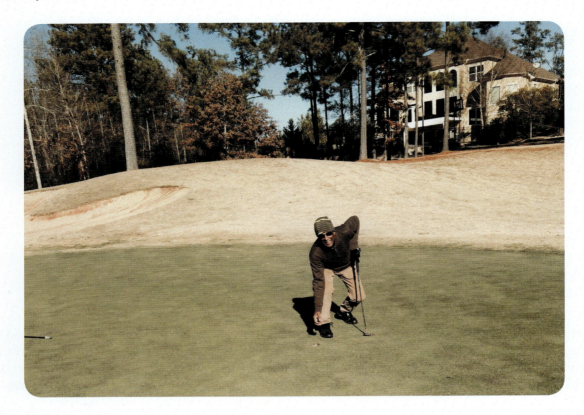

Don had always been a man of purpose, was always helping someone get something done. Whether it was the church communication ministry, serving on the food pantry committee, donating to charity causes (Feed the Hungry, Save the Children), assisting his daughters in stationery design and computer issues, helping his son develop a web page, fixing this and that (remember those birds on my front porch), sharing golf tips and strategies, or offering sage advice, he needed to have something to *do*. He needed purpose. Purpose brought joy into his life, and helping others was his gift. He designed and typeset two of my previous publications, learning new software and consulting with the publisher on a myriad of issues. He designed and assisted with the building of our screened-in porch, an oasis like no other. I Thessalonians 4:11 reads "that you aspire to lead a quiet life, to mind your own business, and to work with your own hands, as we commanded you."

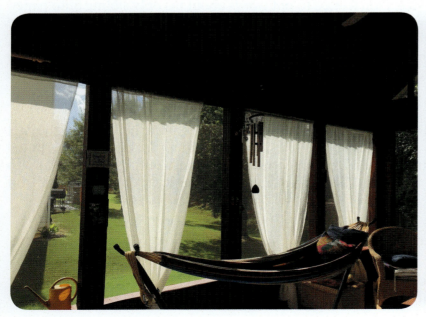

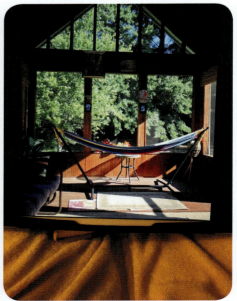

Still, things were not kosher. Don accompanied me on several out-of-town book events when I was marketing *Mashed Potatoes in My Salad: An Alzheimer's Caregiver Journey.* One such event—the South Georgia Literacy Festival in Valdosta, Georgia—had a buffet dinner the night before the festival. As we were passing through the buffet, I was putting food on my plate and Don's when suddenly, he grabbed two big pieces of homemade German chocolate cake from the neatly arranged display, complete with a cake knife, lifted them to his mouth, and began chewing them and licking his fingers at the same time. Please laugh—because I was totally mortified! We immediately returned to our table, where I snatched several table napkins and helped him clean up. Dang! People looked on in horror. I politely informed those at the table and nearby that he was sick and carried on. Yep, his eating habits were not what they used to be. I sensed a meltdown but immediately thought, *We'll never see these folks again, so keep it movin', girlie.* Once again, I embraced my sense of humor in managing whatever this was. By the way, that German chocolate cake was delicious.

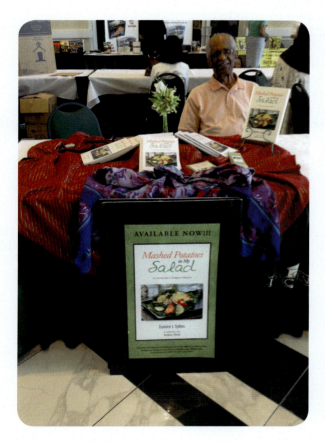

Help me to remember the fruit of the spirit and apply love, joy, peace, patience, kindness, goodness, faithfulness, gentleness, and self-control, for I will need them on this journey (paraphrased, Galatians 5:22).

His mutterings—"Bub . . . bub . . . bub . . . bub . . . bub . . ."—at the beginning of this chapter were the final straw. I suggested he ask his primary care doctor about it. He promised he would. Little did I know he already had some insight. I felt overwhelmed, worried, sad, isolated, and alone, still uncertain of how to manage our lives. I was consumed by his illness, was extremely exhausted from losing sleep, and continued to ignore that tight knot that began its long-term residence in my lower right stomach. I promised myself I would call my doctor and schedule an appointment. I was short on patience, and though I continued golfing, I was withdrawing from other social settings. His doctor's appointment was in two weeks. I couldn't wait.

Please, Lord, let me not be so angry and frustrated. Keep my blood pressure under control. Keep my stomach from churning.

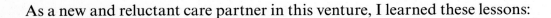

As a new and reluctant care partner in this venture, I learned these lessons:

- Breathe deeply.
- Caregiver burnout is real.
- Check the resource readings from your network (CareNotes, from my church, were awesome).
- Discovery is eye-opening.
- So much depends on the caregiver, who is often tired, frustrated, annoyed, lonely, and impatient.
- Get the most out of the energy you expend.
- Assemble your help team (if only in your mind). The earlier, the better.
- Have a positive approach.
- Examine and be open to respite care options.
- Do not rush your loved one. Slow down, both of you.
- Stay calm.
- Begin to clear your plate. Live more simply.
- Learn to embrace magical moments.
- Be aware of safety concerns.
- Touch your loved one often.
- Share what's happening with other family members, sooner rather than later.
- Handle legal matters while your spouse can make their wishes known.
- Know that this is a time to extend and to receive grace.

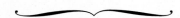

The way forward is to stay hopeful, though for what, I am not sure. As time revealed some of what was coming ahead, I felt like the grips of grieving what we once had had begun. I was nowhere near looking forward to what's next.

CHAPTER 3
The Diagnosis — Mild Cognitive Impairment (MCI), Alzheimer's Disease

This roller coaster ride called mild cognitive impairment . . . I don't think it's Alzheimer's yet. For Don, however, it is the same thing. He's telling people he has Alzheimer's. Whether it's Alzheimer's or any other form of dementia, it is hell.

According to the Alzheimer's Association, mild (early) stage Alzheimer's has similar characteristics to those I describe in the pre-diagnosis chapter. These symptoms have likely been evident for some time and are more pronounced and recognized by people who are in close contact, like a primary care partner. Symptoms often overlap from stage to stage. Loved ones can exhibit a symptom across one or more stages. Prior to diagnosis, Don had been exhibiting all these symptoms:

- Memory loss that disrupts daily life
- Not remembering names when introduced to new people
- Increased trouble with planning and organizing
- Difficulty performing familiar or work-related tasks
- Forgetting material that was just read
- Confusion with time, day, and place
- Trouble understanding visual images and spatial relationships
- New problems with speaking words or writing
- Losing or misplacing valuable objects
- Decreased poor judgment
- Withdrawal from social activities
- Changes in personality

When the primary care physician (PCP) referred us to a cognitive neurologist at a nearby teaching and research health-care facility, it would be two weeks before we could get our first appointment. The session was long and thorough, one part with Don and me, the second part with Don alone.

By the time we got a diagnosis, Don's strange behavior was becoming even more unusual. He still had problems dressing himself, and his personal hygiene was not getting better. Now he often left the garage door up and the inside door to the garage unlocked. Also, by this time, Don could barely write his name or print it. He continued losing weight. When he purchased items over the phone, he would call me to provide the address details to the caller. I was on hyper-alert status, hovering like a helicopter waiting to land. My front-and-center-row seat, with an up-close-and-personal view of this disease, was devastating.

Clearly, when the cognitive neurologist stated that Don had MCI and indicated that there was a fifty–fifty chance of MCI not developing into Alzheimer's, we were hopeful. However, it was not to be. To me, there was nothing mild about the episodes I had witnessed over time. Though this 50 percent chance was not great, at least we had a name and a diagnosis. My simple prayer of gratitude: "Thank you, Lord."

Part of Don's in-depth examination included a mini mental state examination (MMSE), a commonly used, short, credible indicator of cognition loss over time. With scores ranging from zero to thirty, anything less than twenty-six, with the standard score being thirty, is troublesome. Scores less than nine generally indicate severe cognitive impairment, while scores between ten and twenty indicate moderate dementia. Don's score was twenty-two—in the troublesome range. I didn't realize how quickly things could worsen or change. Still primarily ignorant of this disease and its destruction, within a year, Don had full-blown dementia of the Alzheimer's disease type.

Dear God, I don't know what to make of this diagnosis. Help me to be curious, inquisitive, and intelligent in my research, in my walk, in my attitude, in my outlook, in my acceptance of what is to come. In Jesus name.

I began assembling my arsenal of resources. Through my research, I learned the medical profession often has mixed opinions on diagnosing dementia; some doctors do not think a dementia diagnosis changes much.

Here's a quote from a caregiver: "Finally, last year, I asked the neurologist if that (dementia) was what he had; he said, 'I think so.'"

Another said, "The doctors have not been very helpful."

Yet another caregiver reported, "His dementia is undiagnosed. His doctor doesn't think diagnosing will change anything."

The diagnosis is often wrong, unclear, not exact, or labeled mixed dementia. As medications are prescribed by the diagnosis stated, this news was troubling to me. My poem "What Is It?" provides more insight:

So many won't call it out
Some will call out several to be safe
Some will change it as time reveals more
Dementia in any form indicates what is in store

It's going be a long, rough ride
Fasten your seatbelts and watch for the tide
A tumultuous journey—yes, indeed
Prayer, mercy, and grace is what you need.

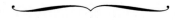

So . . . when are you leaving?

Even before the diagnosis, I believe Don knew he had Alzheimer's. He had too many resources readily available to share with me once he was sure I was on board "through thick and thin, 'til death do us part." During one particular bathroom episode, he voiced defeat. With everything on the table now, he was more certain of me. In the dementia world, once you are diagnosed, you will likely live seven to ten years. We had work to do—living our best lives *better*. Don's beloved saxophone, which I had given to him while we were dating, provided him hours of engagement, relaxation, enjoyment, and activity. My family and I are grateful for those musical moments. Music is so crucial on an Alzheimer's journey.

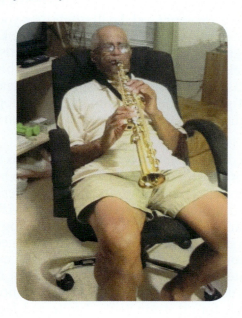

I learned that Alzheimer's disease has a slow decline in memory thinking and reasoning skills (all dementias do) and that Alzheimer's is a fatal disorder, resulting in the loss of brain cells and function. The doctor gave us several prescriptions commonly used for MCI/dementia/Alzheimer's, along with literature to read and digest. That total medicine management thing? It was difficult for both of us. He was taking medicines for his diabetes, cholesterol, and gout, eye drops, a daily aspirin, and now two dementia pills. I was never sure if we did it right. A pill for this, a capsule for that, take one in the morning, another in the evening, two different eye drops with different dosages, not to mention my own pill regimen that I had to manage—honestly, I was never sure.

Don is now not brushing his teeth at night. Sometimes I'm just so tired and frustrated, I don't say anything.

Once our cognitive neurologist visit was complete, we returned to the neurologist, who referred us to a speech therapist. Though it seemed farfetched, we moved forward on that recommendation, hanging, once again, onto some kind of hope. To be candid, with all the ensuing written exercises, the homework assignments, the therapist discussions, and frustrating moments for both of us (I attended each session; by now, I was accustomed to "doing for two"), there was no real improvement in speech for a man who once spoke fluently and extemporaneously and who now had a baffled approach to expressing himself. The therapist also offered a calendar process to help organize Don's days. He was more confused than ever. Her suggestion to post signs around the house were very helpful to Don; they were everywhere, including the refrigerator ("shut door"), the bathroom mirror ("brush teeth," "flush toilet"), and the garage door ("lock door").

It was this female speech therapist on our growing medical team who provided a critical "Aha!" moment of insight to me. As Don struggled through the exercise she guided him through, she glanced at me, saw the tears running down my face, stopped, and shed major light: "Mrs. Sykes, your husband is not having memory issues. He is having *processing issues*." Alzheimer's dementia is not just a memory problem; it is also an information-processing problem, among other things. Think of an iceberg rising out of the ocean. What you see is not what you get. What you don't see is a looming problem. I reflected—ice cream left on the counter all night instead of in the freezer, the desk instructions, the four-pack of tomatoes, and other poor judgment episodes. Indeed, she was right. This discovery made sense to me. Remember that in your journey.

With a clearer understanding of what we were facing, I leaned into a familiar Bible verse: "Fear not. I am with you. Be not dismayed, for I am your God. I will strengthen you. Yes, I will help you" (Hebrews 41:10). Along the way, one of the doctors mentioned clinical trials. Don was eligible (he was taking memory medicines and was diagnosed with MCI). More importantly, he was willing. His thought to make things better for someone else, even if he did not benefit, gave him purpose. Don was hoping for an alternative to "letting the disease run its course." He was eager to learn more by participating to help find treatments and cures. The fighter in him gave him a sense of hope that he was helping research, that memory issues were spotlighted, and that various ethnicities participated in these trials.

Clinical trials are medical procedures designed to answer questions about an investigative medicine to determine if it is safe, if it works, which doses work best, and what the side effects are. We were approved by a local research center. Here he was, an African American, seventy-six-year-old male diagnosed with MCI, offering himself to undergo blood draws, MRIs, PET scans, and spinal taps over ten sessions, some of them overnight, with others beginning at 7:00 a.m., at a location one hour from home. Our thoughts simultaneously went to the Tuskegee Institute and the HeLa blood cells studies where, under dubious and deceitful motives, black people were subjected to medical procedures not in their best interests. Yes, we were skeptical but had nothing to lose. Given the dismal outlook for Alzheimer's and realizing that the trial could not proceed unless I agreed to be a reliable study partner available for all study visits, I followed Don's lead. It was a big decision. Don was willing. So was I. He wanted to fight this disease, to find a cure. His purpose was clear. With this knowledge and no clue of the pending journey and with Don's acceptance and moving forward with the reality that the worst was coming, I mustered up the courage and strength to review all that was before me. Decision fatigue had long ago engulfed me.

> *Be strong and of good courage. Do not be afraid nor be dismayed,*
> *for the lord your God is with you wherever you go.*
> — Joshua 1:9

The clinical trial experience drew us closer together and allowed us to spend relatively uninterrupted quality time together. Car service and a chauffeur were part of the trial perks, and we enjoyed hand-holding and backseat conversation. As I examined death through Don's eyes, he struggled to find words and to read text from magazines. He still enjoyed pictures from golf magazines. He stumbled to get these thoughts out: "Alzheimer's is a horrible disease. It invades your brain and slowly eats away your thinking functions. That's what is happening. Life seems quieter . . . I like the quiet. I can feel your love. I can feel your warm hand, Eunice. I love you. I have said things I should not have said. I was angry, mad, and confused. My world was crashing down on me. I lashed out at you, the one who was there the most. When my time comes, I'll be with old family members—Momma, Pops, Abel, uncles, aunts, cousins . . . Thank you for sharing this life with me."

> *In all things, give thanks, for this is the will of God.*
> — 1 Thessalonians 5:18

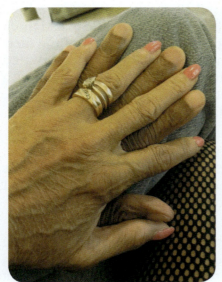

It was about this time that Don shared two books. The first, by Joshua Reynolds, called *20/20 Brain Power: 20 Days to a Quicker, Calmer, Sharper Mind!*, was well underlined, paper-clipped, dog-eared, circled, and notated. The second book, *When Someone You Love Has Alzheimer's*, by Marilynn Larkin, got my attention as it was my first in-depth read into this illness. I was reluctant as I grudgingly gripped the reins of caregiving to an Alzheimer's loved one. This was not the time to have "fight, flee, or freeze" reactions or to be in denial and say, "This is not happening." Don had already done that on his own. While I knew something was off-kilter, I never guessed it was life-threatening. I read both books thoroughly, soaking in the details. Don had insisted I learn how to manage and pay our household bills using our bank account. I was a reluctant student but knew it was essential to ensure everything would be done on time.

He changed his diet to include brain-essential foods like yogurt, salmon, walnuts, ginger, berries, and green tea. He was already taking brisk walks and doing exercises that touted increased brain capacity. He still loved tuna sandwiches from Subway, overflowing with vegetables. He often came home with one sandwich for him and one sandwich for me. I did not love them, but I ate them. He also began cutting back on his favorite alcohol in the purple bag (Crown Royal) and drank red wine instead.

Don felt free to share Alzheimer's-related newsletters and relevant research papers he had ordered from both John Hopkins and Mayo Clinic. He also invited me to visit websites like Lumosity (source: www.lumosity.com), a subscription-based series of brain exercises and games (e.g., puzzles, word finds) designed to strengthen cognitive functioning and decision-making skills. While research is inconclusive on these claims, Don nevertheless enjoyed them while he could.

The best resource he discovered was an introduction to the Alzheimer's Association. This national nonprofit organization became my lifeline. They had a great number of resources, many of them free: literature, educational programs, field trips, social events, volunteers, business cards, and speakers to help and assist. Their support group network (for both caregivers and loved ones with Alzheimer's) was amazing. Overloaded with information, we got involved immediately, even though our local office was an hour away. Monthly, we met others who were on the same path in separate sessions for early-stage dementia loved ones and care partners. I wrote several blogs for their website, using the theme "discovery" to describe this Alzheimer's journey. *Overwhelmed* is another term I often use to talk about dementia. This Bible verse puts things into perspective: "Hear my cry, O God; attend to my prayer . . . when my heart is overwhelmed; lead me to the rock that is higher than I" (Psalms 61:1–2).

The Alzheimer's Association offered business cards for caregivers to use that would discreetly explain that your loved one has Alzheimer's. Preserving your loved one's dignity is so important. These cards are useful in restaurants, when visiting other doctors or dentists or anyone you feel the need to share your loved one's diagnosis with, in any public setting, and at any time (like that cake incident in Valdosta—that would have been perfect). As Don traveled with me to Florida and throughout Georgia to promote my earlier, dementia-related book, I distributed these cards frequently and had no further incidents. I am joyful that he was able to travel with me.

With what little I knew about what was to come, I was definitely not prepared to be a lone caregiver, though it appeared that shouldering the bulk of Don's illness was upon me. He had three adult children, daughters Donna and Kim in California and a son, Don Jr., in Ohio. While their visits were infrequent because of distance, he enjoyed them immensely. I felt alone and isolated and leaned more on my own three children, who were nearby. The midweek "girly" sessions with my daughters, Erica and Nicole, were a refreshing outlet. I looked forward to the respite. My son, Billy, in Florida, checked in regularly and visited when he could.

We switched Don's PCP from one located in Decatur, Georgia, to my PCP located closer to home. The lesson here is to find out the details of all doctor visits to better understand your loved one's history. Please go to the doctor with your loved one so that you can hear and see firsthand what is happening. HIPAA privacy laws may be problematic if you don't.

As I slid into my role as more a reluctant care *partner* than caregiver, I began researching and making a plan; there was no time to feel sorry for myself, worry about house repairs, routine chores, financial matters, car maintenance, or living my life, *our* life. The Don-centered plan emerged. I began to limit scheduling, restrict trips, stay connected with other caregivers (both loving and paid), stay active, stop arguing, go into Don's world, and eliminate stressors. I kept golfing. People often asked if I had planned to or would stop golfing. No, I'd never do that; Don introduced me to golf. I'm holding onto *us*! So I never stopped golfing, though my buddies will say otherwise when I don't play well.

My "Just Do It" T-shirt from the seventies became my mantra. I needed to find and identify more resources. We drew on each other's strength and courage, loved each other, and focused on reclaiming some portion of our lives. That was easier said than done. Common sense told me to take care of myself while taking extra care of Don, to maintain/increase our energy levels, to concentrate on health and vitality, to exercise, and to get plenty of rest. In my head, I knew that to feel refreshed, for whatever amount of time I could carve out, meant I would be better able to care for both of us. I also knew I had to find the good and to be grateful in all things. Knowing this and doing this were two different things. When one is sick, you see, two need help. Within three years, I experienced several health scares as I became more and more engrossed in Don's care and also became an unwilling advocate. The caregiver or partner will need looking after as well as the loved one with dementia. Please take care of yourselves too.

Don was intentional about grooming me for a life without him. He researched and printed numerous articles from the internet relating to Alzheimer's, and I noticed more medical newsletter subscriptions were arriving in the mail. Don shared them with me. He knew well before I did that this was serious. He offered his research findings, which shocked me since I had no idea he suspected his issues were related to dementia. I assumed he had already spoken to his PCP, whom I later discovered also sold Don mind enhancement, your-memory-will-get-better supplements. Be nosy with your loved one's medical team.

Greet one another with a kiss of love.

— 1 Peter 5:14

Help me, Father, to remember Proverbs 17:9. "He who covers a transgression seeks love . . ." In my mind, I know that is so. Help me to live it out when I have anxious and contentious moments.

Many irrational moments led to needless arguments, for I was still learning the lesson of choosing peace over argumentative discussions with "the disease."

Don initially said, "This (Alzheimer's) is not too bad. Cancer or heart problems would be worse."

Two years into the diagnosis, with the previous years of undiagnosed symptoms he'd suffered, he changed his mind. His frustrations continued to mount. I watched him grope for a word, not knowing if I should give it to him. He used his hands when trying to explain something, and he struggled, taking time to get it right. In particular, he could not remember "clouds" and referred to them as "those things in the sky." I often felt sad, irritated, impatient . . . but God! I reminded myself to breathe deeply, to speak softly in short sentences, to look directly at Don when conversing, to go into his world, and to reassuringly touch him often. We often repeated this mantra: "I love you, Don Sykes." "I love you, too, Eunice." Then from us both, it was "It's tough. I know we'll get through it one moment at a time." We seemed to be closing out our spousal relationship to usher in a parent–child relationship. I did not like where we were headed.

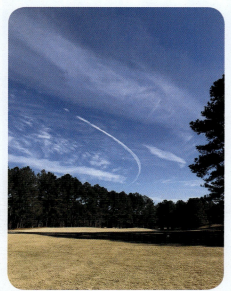

What is this throbbing, lightheaded, swirling sensation I feel in my head? No doubt it's sugar overload, caffeine also. McDonald's sweet tea, no ice, is my drug of choice. Stop it! I've got to do better; I promised myself that.

These times propelled us into decision-making mode. With a diagnosis, we took this opportunity to examine our lives. Don too realized time was not on his side. His new thinking on this disease had shifted.

"It is better to have a hand cut off and be healing than to continually lose my memory and cognitive functioning and have to deal with that."

Though we had plenty of pity parties, we put our affairs in order by educating ourselves, attending local conferences and workshops, identifying support connections and organizations, discussing where he would live, researching long-term living options, deciding driving limitations, and completing the legal paperwork. At Don's suggestion, we visited a lawyer to write a durable power of attorney, living will, advanced directive, health-care directive, financial power of attorney, and update to our will. We remembered the scripture: "Let all things be done decently and in order" (1 Corinthians 14:40).

Since Don was an air force veteran, we made an appointment with the local VA hospital, where Don received additional neurological, psychiatric, and social work visits, nursing home benefits, and a prompt order to stop driving. Without fanfare, that would be his last day of driving a vehicle. We visited the local American Legion as well for Don's socialization and for insights on navigating the cumbersome VA system. One of the social workers told me about a little-known veterans service called aid and attendance benefits, which can supplement financial support for expenses. After a year of tenacious tracking and then completing the paperwork, Don was not eligible. However, it is definitely worth pursuing if your loved one is a veteran and served during the Vietnam War. Another support connection was the Alzheimer's Foundation of America, where I participated in a weekly online support group forum with other caregivers across the nation. I needed and welcomed all the help I could get.

One of the best joy boosters occurred with our connection to the Alzheimer's Atlanta, Georgia, chapter through one of their social events: a black-tie fundraiser called Dancing Stars of Atlanta. We took all day getting ready; I had already learned to slow things down and not to rush a process. My daughters were around to assist and to take pictures—Don, sharp in his black suit (and me in my long red evening gown), socks that matched, starched shirt, cufflinks, clean-shaven, showered, with shoes shined. What a lovely evening! We were among many caregivers and loved ones. It was a magical night for both of us. I felt special and included, without worrying about onlookers noticing Don's behavior. We were all in the same boat. Though the crowd was large, Don felt comfortable. We sat near the door. I relaxed and embraced the fairy tale–like evening . . . that enchanting, joyful moment. I cherished that day and still do; it was the last time Don wore a double-breasted charcoal suit. Doesn't he look *fabulous*?

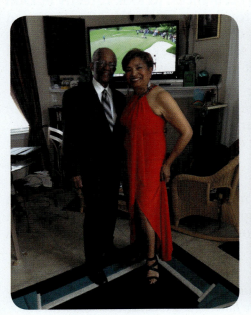 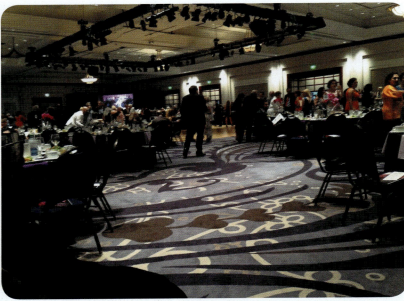

Another poem stirred in my head; I hurried and wrote it on a napkin:

Joy Simmers

It takes up residence.
It lingers.
It rises on occasion.
It's a smile.
It's a nod.
It's a touch.
It's a feeling deep down.
Joy—
O Joy!

The lessons keep coming. They also keep repeating themselves intentionally.

- Alzheimer's is a processing rather than a memory issue.
- This is a hard, long, monumental, arduous, and life-changing journey.

- So much depends on the caregiver, who is often tired, frustrated, annoyed, lonely, and impatient.
- Assemble your help team (if only in your mind). The earlier, the better.
- Have a positive approach.
- Make plans to get away for self-care maintenance.
- Lean on others, whoever they are and wherever they are—your loved ones, your family, your support groups.
- Welcome all input.
- Don't rush. Stay calm. Begin to clear your plate. Slow down. Breathe.
- Learn to embrace magical moments. These are your joy boosters.
- Be aware of safety concerns.
- Touch your loved one often.
- Live more simply.
- Take walks.
- Share your loved one's illness with other family members, sooner rather than later.
- Know that this is a time to receive and to extend grace.
- Get help; the earlier, the better.
- Balance is crucial to you and your loved one.
- It is definitely better to have peace than to be right.
- Pick your battles.
- Prepare to care.
- Short infrequent visits from loved ones will reveal very little of what's going on.
- Strive to be kinder than you feel—always.
- Base tough decisions on your loved one's comfort and not your own.
- Don't worry about how things look; just process how things *feel* to your loved one (and you).

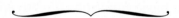

I do know that the way forward is to stay hopeful . . . but for what, I am not sure. As time revealed what was ahead, it felt like the tightening grip of grief over losing my husband and soul mate had already begun. I was devastated and not looking forward to what was next.

CHAPTER 4
Mild (Early) Stage Alzheimer's

For us, the mild (early) stage lasted about two years. The Alzheimer's Association's classic characteristics include the following:

- Personality changes
- Loss of interest in hobbies
- Increased difficulty with usual tasks (e.g., cooking, bill paying)
- Repeated questions and shared stories
- Getting lost
- Hallucinations
- Paranoia
- Mood swings
- Agitation and aggression
- Memory loss and forgetting basic functions (i.e., to eat)
- Weight loss
- Taking other people's things
- Incontinence
- Inappropriate behavior
- Wandering (restless pacing)

While everyone's case is different, it is important to note that not all symptoms occur in sequence and that many of them repeat themselves, perhaps getting increasingly worse from stage to stage. Don was already exhibiting many of these characteristics before his diagnosis. He was still continent, but the inappropriate behaviors continued. For instance, somehow my microwave stopped fully heating food in the middle of the glass plate turntable. We'd had a spaghetti episode; my guess was that Don must have put a metal pot in the microwave to heat the spaghetti as it had seemed to explode, the contents of which were also all over the stove. He obviously was trying to fix himself a plate of food, but the inexplicable could have happened, and he was trying to clean it up. His wandering was also ongoing throughout the disease.

He uses his hands a lot and makes gestures to help me figure what he wants to say. Or says it finally after seconds or minutes. He feels bad that he doesn't get it out when he wants.

We'd play our own personal game of charades, it seemed. Though Don's lapses in conversation or the same conversation occurred repeatedly, he was speaking his mind much better, mixing words and sounds that made up our conversation. His daily three-mile walks through the neighborhood were coming to an end, as were his trips to the gym and to the music store. His perception issues made him prone to falling, with an unsteady gait. In fact, he'd already had two falls: coming down the stairs at home and then at the golf course, getting out of the golf cart. I worried constantly if he might open the door and walk outside. Safety was foremost in my mind. Jokingly, I now thought of him as "Don with a side of dementia." Sadly, it was more like *dementia, with Don locked inside.*

The aluminum trash can liner lid was gone too, probably out with the weekly trash. My mother's treasured dish was shattered, his missing wedding ring was likely buried in the yard, the checking account was overdrawn, creditors were sending notices, and the toilet areas reeked with waste that missed the mark. The same questions repeated like a mantra: "What time is it? Where are we going? When are we leaving?" He was unable to count backward. However, he still watched and enjoyed golf, played his horn, worked in the yard, drank wine, and made his bed, military style. I preached this lesson to myself halfheartedly, "With the good, the bad, and the ugly of Alzheimer's, keep it all in perspective and move forward, one step at a time, one moment at a time."

"I know how to go, but I can't tell you." What did that feel like to Don? Exasperating for him.

We see good scenery.

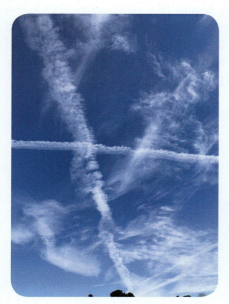

When I drove him places, he loved to observe the environment. Water was his reference to the clouds in the sky, knowing that rain came from them. He never again said the word *clouds*. His golf game was off as he chose the wrong clubs: he'd taken a putter to the fairway and a driver for his second shot, aimed the club in the opposite direction, and didn't strike the ball like he once did.

When we got to the green, he asked, "Where is the hole? I'm at the hole holding the flag."

He did not understand. I remembered these words from the speech therapist again: "It's a processing issue, not a memory problem." We moved on. With his golf crew, he'd lost several clubs, including a putter. There were extras in the garage, yet he spent $150 to buy another. How do you lose a putter? Easily! Just ask my beloved Don.

Don is often confused. He goes into the kitchen looking for soup on the stove . . . he cannot figure it out. "Where's the stove? Where's the soup?" Looks at the counter on the opposite wall. What is it that keeps me solidly planted while all things around me are falling apart, going haywire? My soul is anchored in the Lord. Though the storm keeps on raging in my life. Thanks be to God for the songwriter Thomas Whitfield. My staple since the 80s. The song? "My Soul's Been Anchored."

With immense challenges still ahead, along with daunting tasks, Don's confusion and worsening symptoms were glaring; there were times when our home utilities were cut off because of the lack of payment, like the time the water bill was overdue and the water company had shut off the supply. It was like living in a Third World country or, closer to home, like the Flint, Michigan, water fiasco. He began spitting. Nightly, Don played his soprano saxophone but often returned it to the horn case the wrong way or laid it down rather than upright in the horn holder. My daughter Nicole and grandson Nicholas have fond memories (without all the drama) of hearing him nightly, playing his "sexy sax" as they would approach the front door.

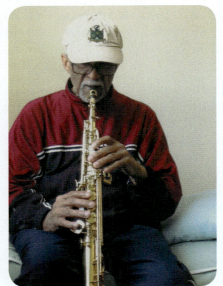

It's a "brown sock, blue sock" kind of day.

I began closely monitoring Don for ADLs or activities of daily living. His hygiene habits had changed—bathing, brushing teeth, applying deodorant and lotion to his body, distinguishing soap from lotion, properly putting on clean clothes, pulling a golf shirt onto his leg, and eating when I was gone. He often appeared in his underwear as he'd lost much of his inhibitions and watched television all day. Sometimes he blew his horn. He no longer spent as much time in his upstairs office. When he did though, he still went up the stairs without using the hand rails.

We cruised to the Bahamas for four days with some difficulty. Smaller rooms, toilets flushing differently, and tiny showers further confused Don. Coming home, we had a twelve-hour layover in Orlando, Florida, which tired both of us. He went to the bathroom in one entrance and came out another entrance and was lost for half an hour; I spent a harrowing thirty minutes with the airport security tracking him down. In an area with six ramps around a food court circle, things could have been much worse. I was so thankful that episode ended well, though my nerves were completely shot. Shortly after, I discovered the Alzheimer's Association offered the "Help! I've Fallen!" button, which we promptly wore from that point on, along with our med alert and ID bracelets. What a joyful, timely gift!

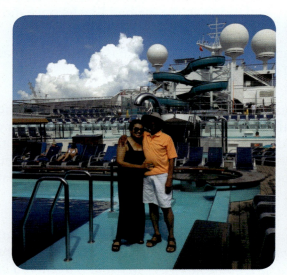

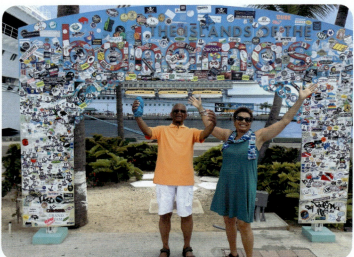

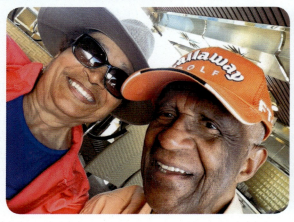

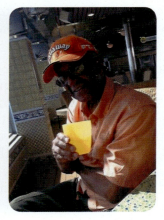

The doctors are doing all they can.

On Easter Sunday, as we returned home from church, Don asked, "What is Calvary?"

Heartbreaking? Indeed. For Christians around the world, Calvary is central to the Easter story. It is the location of the cross where Jesus was crucified. These continual circumstances led to our first respite experience at an adult day care. We went to several sites together until I got smart and left him home after a particular visit. It was better to have an uninterrupted, focused visit so I could tolerate the rates being quoted without screaming. Expenses for care are not cheap! His MMSI scores continued to drop, indicating both disease progression and my need for additional help.

In the conference room, where we checked in for registration at our first respite stay, the loving and attentive staff (Don wanted black caregivers; theirs was a diverse team) asked me questions such as "Are you stressed? Tired? Frustrated?"

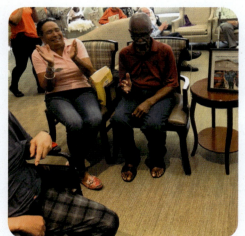

Before I could answer, Don replied, "All of the above."

We all laughed—the intake nurse, Don, and me.

I'm feeling weary; he's feeling weary.

That was the truth! I was also exasperated, beat down, unhinged, crazy, seething, and paranoid. You may have noticed these are also traits of a loved one with dementia. We were both frayed at both ends, like the rope that I kept in the backseat of my car throughout this journey, which represented the jostling of our lives. Often, while I nervously peeled dry skin from my hands until they ached, Don bit and chewed his fingernails. We were both "nervous Nellies." A dear family friend said it best: "Love the one taking care of the loved one." She was right; doing for two was killing me.

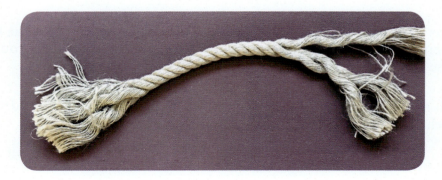

He wants to be my hero; he is my hero. He wants to be helpful. He is sometimes. Other times, I would rather do things myself.

Once we acted on our decision, I dropped Don off at seven thirty and picked him up at four thirty three times per week. He was happy making new friends, interacting with the staff, and helping out where he could (that purpose thing again).

"What can I do to show thanks? You like that? Let me have the other one."

When the nurse on duty suggested Don give me a foot rub, he remembered. While watching TV, he reached down, got my right foot, and proceeded to rub my leg and foot. I let him finish and went to the other side so he could rub my left foot too!

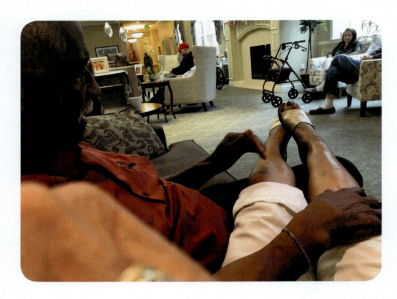

"I try my best to get along with you, and this is what I get . . ." In a while, he will have forgotten what he said.

Within three weeks, paranoia reared its ugly head. Don had several "mean" days. The disease was in full control. His fighting spirit was in gear the wrong way.

He ranted on the way home: "You have seen how f****d up things are in that place . . . I can't do nothing. I want to be with you and do some things! People don't have to do s**t for me! I am gonna find a way to change this! I try to do my best. I bust my ass for s**t every night! I try my best!"

The disease was definitely in charge with this tirade. He was visibly upset as he walked—no, *stomped*—the circle from our keeping room to the kitchen, to the dining room, through the hallway, into the living room, and back.

I let him finish and smilingly said, "You're right," and walked into the bedroom. I'd finally modified my behavior. Yes. It is better to have peace than to be right.

He's tired, I can tell . . . disgusted, mad, angry.

On one other occasion, he said, "I don't want to be with these old folks. They are old."

His sense of humor, who he was, was still intact. Every day was an adventure. I am overjoyed, still today, when I reflect on this memory.

"Yes . . . You're right, babe."

"You are the best thing that's ever happened to me."

I recognized Don was soon headed to a different kind of long-term living arrangement as I took him to adult day care daily and the costs were climbing. With this in mind, we built more memories. We went to a jazz festival in Panama City, Florida. Letting love lead the way, we created joyful memories that sustained us throughout his illness and, even now, still for me. Take a look!

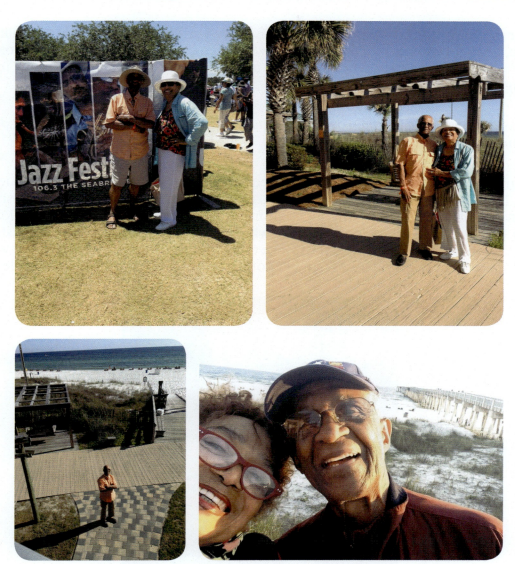

Winter came and went. We spent New Year's in Florida, visiting extended family.

My daughter Erica picked a good, calm time to tell me, "Mom, people are noticing you look very tired . . ."

We missed several Sundays of worship; one of his concerned friends called to check on us.

I was sure to tell him, "We are moving slower these days."

When Don recognized his milk was already poured on his cereal after going to the refrigerator to get it, he was puzzled when he said, "That ain't good, what I just did."

I replied, "Nope, it ain't good, but at least you recognized it."

His reply: "I know . . . I'm forgetting that I forgot." Powerful statement.

It was clear that I was the most important person in his world. How did I feel about that? I had to focus more, be in the moment more, enjoy him while I could. I hadn't expected our golden years to be like this. We laughed at that joyful boost and strove to be happy and flourish in times of great change.

He wants to know when my birthday is . . . It's been on his mind. Worries he'll forget. Asks for help putting it on his calendar.

Don's family from California visited for a week. Don was delighted to spend time with his daughters, Donna and Kim, and grandson Marc. When his eldest niece, Dawn, came, she enjoyed beautiful moments on the patio singing "Summertime," while Don played the melody on his saxophone. She even released me for a day to do whatever I wanted. I wrote a note suggesting things she might do with him. This gave me some respite time, which I sorely needed. Now *that* was a good show of support! I am thankful for her and her other acts of kindness during her uncle's illness.

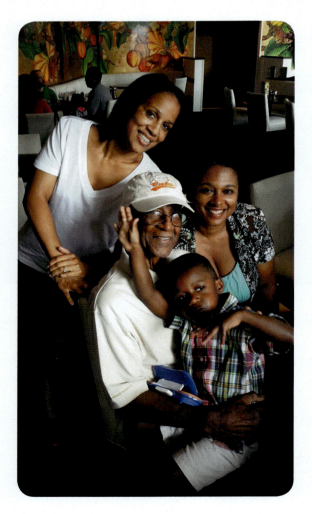

Other family members as well as our church family visited during this time. I was able to complete a 5K fundraiser race for Alzheimer's and spoke locally on the subject. I also kept a blessing jar containing my own weekly uplifting positive messages to be read as needed.

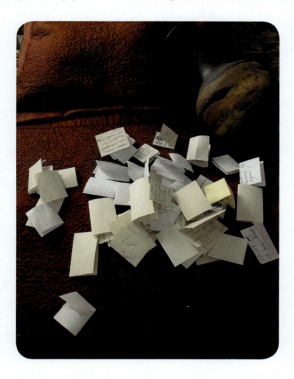

Near summer's end, after one Bible study meeting where Don took copious notes (one was "God, show me the purpose of my life") in the margins of his Bible with highlighted specific verses, he looked at me and said, "I'm not getting better. Make sure I am taken care of."

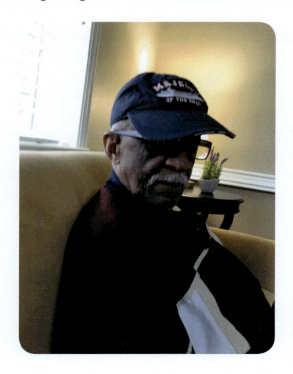

Lessons learned are the following:

- Be thankful. Develop an attitude of gratitude.
- Be realistic about what you can handle.
- Go into their world.
- Don't rush; take your time.
- Pick your battles.
- Maintain your own health; keep your doctor appointments.
- Exercise and get plenty of rest.
- Get your paperwork, legal and financial, done.
- Pat yourself on the back. You're doing okay. You'll be okay.
- Take drives and walks.
- Make photo albums for your loved one.
- Flip through a picture book of family (Don loved that and would identify people I didn't know).
- Eat an apple.
- Watch golf, if applicable; do your loved one's favorite things.
- Take deep breaths.
- Enjoy peaceful, quiet time outdoors.
- Keep a blessing jar and fill it with one positive statement weekly; read them as necessary.
- Uncertainty interacting with loved ones transcends all stages. Get help.
- Making changes in life means making changes in you.
- Wherever you are in your journey, connect with others who are also caring for loved ones.
- Don't take things personally. Mood and attitude changes are part of this disease.
- Most episodes involve a processing issue, not a memory issue.
- Vow to live your best life *better* despite Alzheimer's.
- Accept what you cannot change; you've made the best decisions.
- Give yourself some grace.
- It is better to be at peace rather than right.
- Increase self-care.
- Mild hearing loss contributes to dementia; schedule an appointment sooner rather than later.

I still believe that the way forward is to stay hopeful . . . but always hopeful for *what* exactly? I am not sure. As time continued to reveal what was coming ahead, I felt like the grip of grief was ongoing, had accelerated, and was escalating. I was not looking forward to what was next.

CHAPTER 5
Long-Term Care

"I want to go somewhere to live, night and day."

For many people, long-term care is not an option. It is not a solution, whether they have had discussions with their loved ones who voiced adamant disagreement about going somewhere else to live or whether they can even access the finances for such an expensive option. It is expensive. For others who can work through the maze of finances, types of housing available, and wishes of the loved one with appropriate input from others, long-term care can be an acceptable choice among choices. One statistic to consider is that often the ratio of paid staff to patients in long-term facilities is eight to one; at-home care is less than that. It seemed logical to me that eight people with eyes trained on your loved one, who also cared for them, was a good thing. Even a four-to-one ratio was better than me primarily handling all the necessary caretaking tasks. There was much work to be done, and the duties would only get heavier. Another primary consideration for me to consider was if something happened to me and I began to cave under the caregiver load, who would take care of Don?

We considered long-term care insurance years before this disease entered our lives but didn't find it useful for us for several reasons. The primary reason was the high cost versus the benefits; they were not worth the premiums. Even Don's employer, where he'd been for twenty years, had group rates that were not reasonable. For us, this option was going to be an out-of-pocket expense. I sharpened my pencil as I considered where I was going to find the funds. It was time to finagle finances. All my life, I had been a good steward of my finances; now was the time to work my magic. I examined closely every item in our budget.

Senior living advisor referral and placement services connected to partner resident communities are readily available to families seeking assistance. These organizations are reimbursed by partner communities. They offer screening services that narrow your visit choices with questions such as "Is your loved one's short-term memory repetitive?" Yes. "Does he wander?" Yes . . . especially if he were in a strange place; he would look for me. "Is he completely independent in walking? Is he ambulatory?" Yes and yes. Depending on what stage you are in with your loved one's dementia, there are many options for getting help. My goal for long-term alternate living was to find a safe, secure environment for Don to explore his remaining independence. Both the care and the rent varied, and a resident assessment is always required before admission. All of them are expensive. I considered care within the home and care outside of the home, including adult day care, companion care, personal care, short-term care, nursing homes, skilled nursing facilities, family group homes, board and care facilities, and long-term assisted living, with or without memory care.

Once Don's early-stage episodes became more frequent and nerves on both sides became frayed and tattered, he brought up the subject of living elsewhere several times over several months. He was clear from the beginning too that his caregivers should be African American, preferably males. His discussions removed most of the guilt associated with living elsewhere. Starting early made the admission process much easier once the decision was made. So we pursued this option, knowing that this was going to be a financial challenge. Don passed the front door many times during the day and night to come upstairs. His wandering and sleeplessness (and my sleeplessness) became a safety factor since he had also fallen several times on the stairs. More and more, he was becoming unable to function on his own. Seldom was he aggressive, but in one angry outburst, Don slammed the car door in the driveway, threw his books and his jacket to the ground, and proceeded walking toward a nearby state highway. Overwhelmed, I needed help caring for him. We moved forward, considering many issues: the physical age, design, and appearance of the building; the pricing structure; the residents' care and appearance, the number of staff and their qualifications; recommendations from others; and memory care focus. Typically, I visited sites first for a look-see and then brought Don, if appropriate. "Tour plus lunch" was the usual model, though I often just "dropped in."

A facility specializing in Alzheimer's care located in Morrow, Georgia, was my first foray into optional living arrangements. Someone in my network had used them in the past and recommended them highly. My near-term goal: respite care. This particular assisted living facility was a well-hidden, well-kept secret for those with memory issues and their caregivers. Personal assistance-provided services included bathing, grooming, toileting, transportation, meal preparation, dressing, medicine management, socialization, and companionship in a safe, respectful, and compassionate manner.

After being buzzed in (all doors remained locked), I was greeted by a friendly, professional staff, all of whom were African American. I learned that this state-licensed facility was an "adult day care," with drop-off times before 9:00 a.m. and with a pickup time in the evening no later than 5:00 p.m. Overnight stays and weekend services were limited. Their goal was to provide respite to caregivers and to give loved ones a meaningful, productive, engaging environment, complete with breakfast, lunch, and an afternoon snack. Costs were relatively reasonable and based on a sliding scale. I was impressed, while Don wandered through the building. That was a good thing. We completed the paperwork, and Don was approved. He loved his stay at this facility; he spent a year there, more time than I planned. The cost of care there was fast approaching the cost of long-term memory care with overnight accommodations. I remembered Don was, in fact, in an adult day care facility, not an overnight facility. Something had to give.

An interim solution came through our VA social worker connections, who shared that veterans benefits included a free thirty-day stay at an approved nursing home. We chose a facility close to downtown. Services provided were meaningful engagement activities and overnight accommodations in a single room, with daily breakfast, lunch, and dinner and a snack as well as medicine management, routine weighing, blood pressure, and pulse checks. This service allowed me time to identify, research, and complete due diligence on several options in the area within fifty miles. I recommend selecting a facility that is not close to your home so that you can plan and schedule your visits appropriately. Gut feelings and what the staff are doing when you "drop by" are more important than the age and type of facility you are considering. I also recommend a facility that is on one level. Also, identify the contact information on the local ombudsman who will assist you if there are problems/concerns that are not handled satisfactorily with management. I completed a mountain of paperwork, and Don was admitted and stayed the entire thirty days. The amazing social worker there also assisted me in deciding the proper facility for Don's long-term care; she confirmed that he was not yet ready for permanent placement in a nursing home.

"You will see to it that I am taken care of . . ."

There's that gentle instruction again. Meanwhile, after fourteen visits (without Don) to places all over Atlanta, I narrowed the search to two south-side locations where the staff was diverse, friendly, and helpful and the one-floor building design was in a rectangular traffic flow. My decision was made. As it was near the end of the month, I was able to negotiate a lower rate than was originally quoted, and I could use my "cash back" credit card for his monthly payment. That Monday, with five days rent free and one suitcase, Don and I traveled to his new home, a long-term memory care facility located twenty-five miles from my home, where he would live for the next two years.

This brings me to the guilt associated with considering having around-the-clock care or interim care to supplement and complement your care. Don't allow your spouse or any loved one to make you feel guilty, even if they oppose help. No one knows the toll this disease takes on everyone involved. *Take care of you.* If you need help, get help. Period. Since Don, in the earlier stages of his disease, brought up long-term living arrangements, my guilt was eased, guilt was eased. In any case, I was happy to investigate. Here are the advantages I found. Again, caregiver staff in these facilities often number eight to one; any number is better than one, you alone. Paid caregivers often are more capable with dealing with episodes and better equipped to handle your loved one. Many of them love what they do. They help to get you out of the way. When your loved one is settled in their new surroundings and they want to come home, seek out the paid staffer help to intervene, deflect, and divert your loved one. Speak to your doctor regarding adjusting your loved one's medicines. Stay on top of what's happening and speak up when necessary.

Don and I moved forward with these additional lessons learned:

- Begin your research on long-term care options early.
- Long-term facilities often have waiting lists for accommodations.
- Show up at your loved one's facility regularly and at odd times.
- Never say never.
- Get to know the staff.
- Find an internal friend.
- Visit facilities to observe.
- Choose to remember more with love than with pain.
- Stay vigilant; if you see something, say something.
- Don't second-guess your decisions; lean where you need to lean.

CHAPTER 6
Moderate (Middle) Stage Alzheimer's

For us, the moderate (middle) stage of Alzheimer's lasted about four years.

Classic characteristics from the Alzheimer's Association include an increase in symptoms previously mentioned and others:

- Increased forgetfulness
- Feeling moody or withdrawn in most settings
- Unable to recall personal information (e.g., high school attended, birthday, place of birth)
- Confusion about recent conversations, location, current day
- Required help with clothing choices
- Toileting habits worsen, double incontinence
- Getting lost and wandering
- Being argumentative
- Hallucinations
- Paranoia
- Increased irritability, anxiety, and depression
- Sleep disturbances
- Hand wringing, tissue shredding
- Falls
- Spoken sounds or an inability to verbally communicate pain
- Hospice considerations

This stage is typically the longest; it was for Don. He required a greater level of care. He was consistently losing weight. His appetite, still, was good; I used food cueing to encourage him to eat, which he often did with his hands. I could no longer leave him during the day. He was up walking the house most of the night. If I was in another room, he came looking for me ("shadowing"). I was always mindful that he would likely walk past our front door with three locks and out into the streets. This is called "wandering" in the Alzheimer's world, though for a time, I just considered it "walking off" energy. He wandered throughout his illness.

For me, dementia (specifically Alzheimer's) is the worst disease in the world. As I attempted to keep my body, mind, and spirit fresh, I could not, in all sincerity, manage my issues along with everything else. I knew the time had come to allow space for and give to myself grace. My documented videos, photos, phone calls, and observations over time were overwhelming though educational and delightful all at the same time. This shedding and clearing of my mind—putting my experience to paper, on the desktop computer, iPhone, iPad, or wherever I could unload— was my grace. My personal and intimate journey through Alzheimer's did not need a "virtual experience" to find out how cruel and unforgiving the path this disease takes through the lives of your loved ones and their family caregivers. Our relationship was definitely no longer a spousal or even a partner liaison. Indeed, it was that of a caregiver or mother–child venture. I remember twice, I tried to do the virtual experience, a series of lifelike encounters that mimic living with Alzheimer's. I quit at the third juncture because it was real time. It was quite upsetting. My reality was unsettling enough.

Dear God, sometimes I think it's me that has the problem. That I am the person with the sick brain. Ha! Woe to both of us if I get sick. Keep me, Jesus. In His name.

Two years before Don entered memory care, my own health issues began to surface, raising more urgency to get him placed. Three health scares took precedence as I was Don's sole caregiver and had little time to concern myself with my symptoms. Yes, it is important to stay healthy. I had to confront a nagging, consistent pain in my lower right stomach, head-swirling sensations, a ringing in my ears, and an abnormal annual mammogram. Again, I knew that if I got sick, no one would be able to take care of Don and his increasing progression in the manner required. I was also dipping into my personal retirement savings to handle the added expenses.

I was headed nonstop toward classic caregiver burnout, while Don's symptoms of moderate stage Alzheimer's, aside from those mentioned earlier, were increasing:

- Personal hygiene assistance with bathing and brushing teeth
- Balancing issues
- Increased falls, resulting in repeated head trauma, brain bleeding, and brain cells dying
- More confusion
- Difficulty swallowing
- Tremors (slight for Don, on his right hand)
- Constipation
- Slight cold
- Incontinence
- Toileting schedule (every two hours)
- Appropriate bedding and undergarments
- Calling me "Momma" and misidentifying or not recognizing other family members

"This stuff is getting worse. The things I used to do, I can't do."

Don, thoughtful one morning after a particularly bad previous day, turns toward me and haltingly says, "I want to talk to you . . . Yesterday made me realize all the things I can't do. I just don't have it. I was hoping I could beat this thing. Obviously, I can't. You will make sure I am taken care of. You do what's best. I am sure you are doing all the best things to do. I was thinking I was gonna get rid of this. It ain't gonna happen."

"I got your back," I say.

"I know you do. It's not changing. It's not gonna get any better. I keep f***ing up. I am not making any improvements on what's happening. Still hopeful for a cure. Until then, I gotta deal with what it

is. Sykes, it's not working. It's over, man. Who knows? The Lord might say, 'I got something for you, Sykes.' But it's taking a long time."

Don acknowledged having suicidal thoughts and wanting to die. On our last visit to the VA, the doctors pronounced him clinically depressed (I'm sure I was too). It took weeks to get a referral. Meanwhile, the doctor asked if I had weapons around our home and recommended that, if so, I should hide them. I did. He also suggested I confirm our fire alarms worked. I did.

"I want to go somewhere to live night and day."

It was with these current and looming concerns that we moved forward on our joint decision to enter a newly opened memory care, long-term assisted living facility. I visited this particular place a year earlier as part of my due diligence and found it too expensive. I told them that their rates were higher than the surrounding market. Yes, they had a new building to pay for—but not at my expense! This time, they offered special rates with the current month's five remaining days free. I committed after four years of a nonstop, 24/7-type caregiving. I negotiated using a "cash back" credit card, creating a small income stream. Did you get that important detail? Know that you can negotiate rates.

Finished VA paperwork, third time around, for help with long-term assisted living.

By this time, Don's MMSE score had dipped to ten. We needed help. I had three surgeries, with follow-up care and time to recuperate ongoing. While I waited to hear from the VA on the status of our aid and attendance application (it was ultimately declined), once more, I finagled finances as best I could, and God provided a workable solution. Don was both excited and upset to move. I packed enough clothes for a week's stay, and we were off and running for this new experience. Before I left the facility, Don wandered off in his new safe surroundings with locked entrances and began socializing with others. I was delighted. My to-do list included handling more paperwork, scheduling a current tuberculosis shot (we used a convenient mobile TB unit; it was the weekend), gathering his medical records and his medication schedule, and creating a "life snapshot" document, a narrative of who he was, so that the staff could get to know him. I enjoyed putting that together, with his input. His life was full of living.

Though this time was an "up and down" experience with many "Aha!" moments, it was the best decision for us. I knew that. After dropping Don off on his first day, I sat in the parking lot, and my dam of tears was opened. It was the "ugly cry," one that had been building over time. I was shivering, heaving, and banging the steering wheel. I took my time; I needed this! I knew this was the right solution for us, yet I was still torn. I did not experience guilt, however. I also vowed again to shed my not-so-healthy obsession of choice—sweet caffeinated tea, no ice, preferably from McDonald's. Minutes later, I pulled out of the lot and went home. I was happy that Don was safe, comfortable, and cared for. I looked forward to nights without sleep interruptions and dates with my husband at museums, restaurants, and parks, lunch at one of our favorite spots (Kentucky Fried Chicken), malls, support group meetings, and even doctor appointments.

Over time, two of the biggest issues of concern were UTIs and foot fungus. Don contracted both. He regularly had flu shots and had the sniffles on occasion but never a cold. An active advocate now, I discovered that sharing my knowledge of Alzheimer's was helpful to the staff. For example, I often shared proper hands-on arm techniques when touching loved ones and upcoming education events throughout the city. Someone along the way gave me a hands-on resource loaded with fun, stimulating, seasonal activities designed to make the time with a loved one productive and stimulating called "A Year Together: Activities for Persons with Alzheimer's Disease." I shared it with the activities director, who held a crucial role for engagement activities within the community. I also created a photo album of Don's nuclear family—which included his mom and dad, uncles and aunts—to stimulate his long-term memory and supplemented his admittance paperwork with anecdotes related to his personal history, such as work, hobbies, health history, and family ties. It, along with three other family photos I created on Shutterfly, were well used throughout Don's stay. Don attracted people. He celebrated two birthdays with his new family.

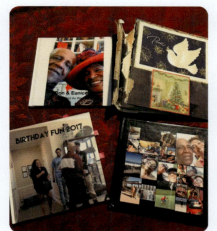

I held his hand as he turned seventy-nine, noting, "We're still here, babe!"

He enjoyed the evening with wine and cheese.

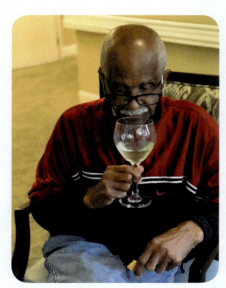

His lifetime love of dancing was evident as music stirred his soul. He was uninhibited at the sound of music and enjoyed the fellowship and companionship within the community and with the residents' loved ones who visited. The residents were loving, kind, and engaging. Many were lonely. I noticed some residents had few visitors. Others had no visitors. I spent time getting to know and loving on them. They blessed me. Meanwhile, Don eagerly participated in the daily activities, which included singing, standing and chair exercises, group play, bowling, checkers, live entertainment, and worship. Don especially loved the musicians, listening, grooving, and clapping his hands to such tunes as "Mustang Sally," "Knock on Wood," "Turn Back the Hands of Time," and "Get Down Tonight." We often danced like no one was watching. Don took over the floor, swinging, snapping his fingers, and clapping while remaining stable on his feet.

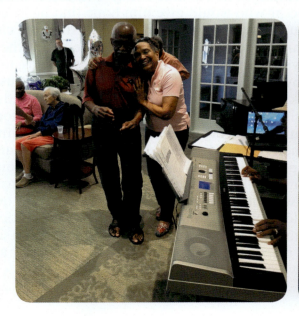 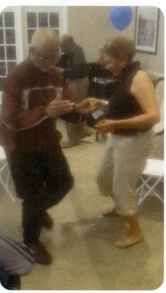

We also slow-danced. Don's love of dancing—I mean, *really* dancing—surfaced again and again during his Alzheimer's journey. Our slow dances were joyful and special. With solid, comforting, familiar hands near the small of my back, Don would lead me into our dance, our space . . . We'd sway gently, slowly, and steadily into a place where there would be just the two of us. We could both close our eyes for a moment. I beamed; he beamed. What a reminder of what was . . . and still is. Our love remains—a joyful, boosted moment.

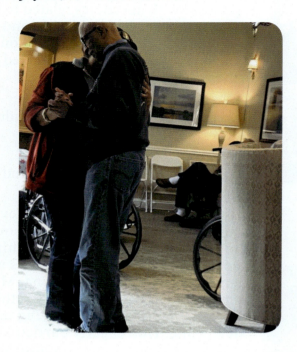

Eventually, we personalized his very own shadow box, which hung on the wall outside his suite. For months, he did not have a roommate, though he occupied a double-bedroom suite. We shared great one-on-one time in a new setting, with help just outside the door. Oh, the joy that flooded my soul! I was his wife again and was ecstatic about dating my husband.

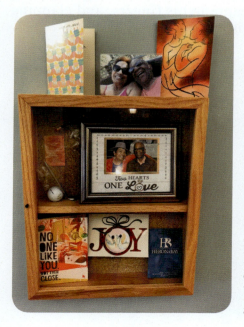

In the days and months ahead, Don settled into a routine. Interestingly, he equated being in assisted living with seeing a doctor who would give him hope that he would get better. Though his sleep patterns (or lack thereof) changed little, he thrived while participating in the life of the community: enjoying group exercises, making new friends, joking with the happy and friendly staff, eating three delicious meals and a snack (I sometimes ate with him), getting his meds on schedule, dancing with the residents, and playing his saxophone (which I would then bring home nightly). When I left things behind at this new place, I discovered they would disappear. We adopted one particular staff member as his caring companion; his comment, "Don's a fighter!" let me know his insights into my man were on point. He and Don seemed to click quickly. I hired him for a birthday-and-all-other-things celebration event at my community. His job was to be Don's companion sitter, while we both enjoyed our friends and family from near and far. What an awesome joyous memory, even today!

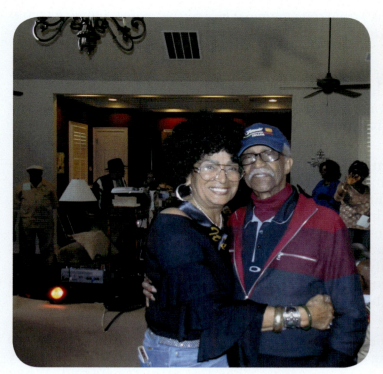
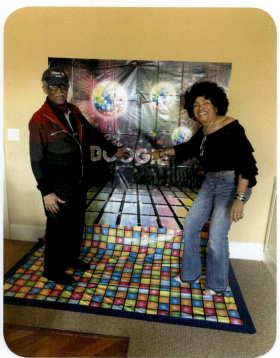
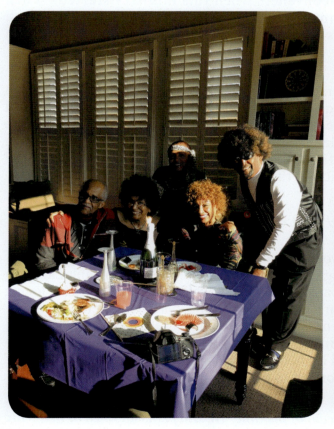
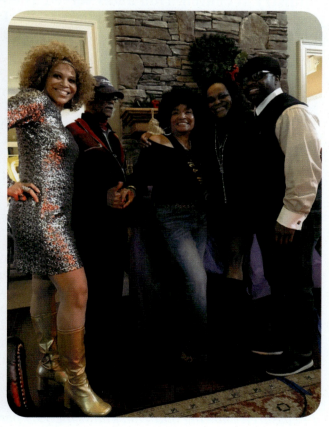

We enjoyed each other in whatever way we could. I often read from a meditations book, personalizing the message just for Don. He would engage and smile as he walked toward me. When well-intentioned and loving visitors remarked that they were unsure of how to interact with Don, I suggested this meaningful, joyful activity.

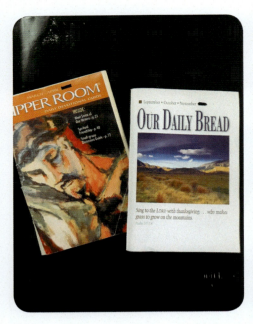

He asks from time to time if he's getting worse. I think he is but instead say, "Babe, you're holding your own."

Other times, Don would walk off, going into his consistent wandering habit by pacing in his controlled environment. He was living *his* best life better in spite of the Alzheimer's progression being ever present.

Eventually, a roommate was assigned briefly to Don's room; I objected. Added issues with bodily fluids, toileting, clothing, bathing supplies, personal hygiene items, shavers, toothpaste, and toothbrushes scared me. I objected again, and within a short period, they were separated. I already knew that Don was not always in control of his bodily functions, that he had accidents and then would be apologetic, easing tension in the moment. I did not need another person in the mix.

I continued my self-care rituals and tried to maintain a schedule (isolation is not good; be intentional about socializing), including one of my favorites: attending the married couples ministry at church. Don and I served as co-conveners when this ministry started. When members joined and introduced themselves, I introduced Don, showing his picture on my cell phone. If I was present, he was present. Here's a picture of lovebirds we painted (Don's is on the left):

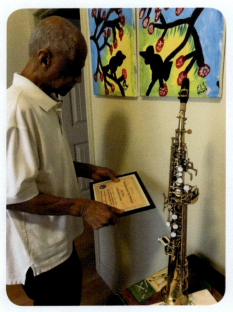

My northern trips to my support group activities also continued. I quickly realized the benefits of having a spousal group on the south side, where we lived, and formed the Southside Alzheimer's Spousal Support Group. Five people attended the first meeting, acknowledging the lonely and tired trek of devotion to their loved one.

"You need help? Do you need help with anything?"

One of my favorite dates with Don was at a nearby par-three golf course. Though his game was off, he was comfortable carrying the bag and walked the grounds while I played. Alongside loving wife, I took on new roles as a loving, persistent, fierce advocate, overseer, and monitor. My sleeping patterns got better, though I was functioning on less than five hours nightly and my anxiety level was still high. My doctor prescribed a take-the-edge-off pill. It is important to get as much rest as you can.

I'm assured knowing that Don knows me 99.9 percent of the time. He still perks up when he hears my "Hey, babe!" greeting, either over the phone or in person.

When I visited (with no set schedule; loved ones had keys to enter), Don recognized my "Hey, babe!" voice, turned in my direction, greeted me with that twinkle in his eye when he realized I was there, and gave me big, loooooong (yes, spelled as they felt), warm hugs. As we embraced,

I could feel his body relax. I held him until he let go. He grabbed my briefcase or backpack as we walked the hallways. What an awesome, joyful boost! No arguments and contentious energy in the air—instead, we enjoyed a pleasant evening with each other in a calming, home-like setting. These were times to replenish, restore, and rejuvenate my caregiver's soul.

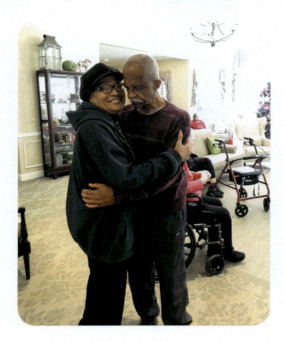

My grandson Kory came often to cut his "pop-pop" Don's hair. Don would never let anyone else get that close to his face. He enjoyed the attention. Kory enjoyed these moments too. What a joyful boost!

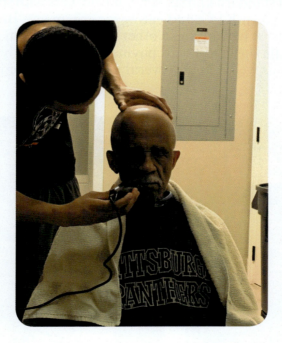

We spent our togetherness with love. We held hands, he rubbed my shoulders and legs, and we looked intently at each other. We smiled at each other. We talked about family he grew up with and other people in his photo albums. His smile was the biggest sign that he knew they were special. What a joyful boost!

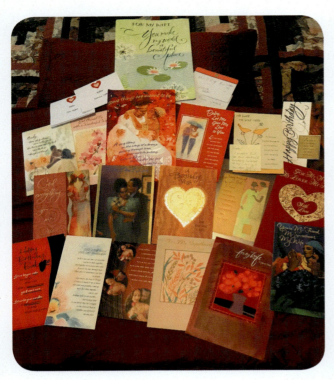

When I was not there, Don called me often. If I was unable to answer, he left cryptic voice messages that are still on my cell phone and that I still listen to. My delight in these joyful moments keeps me, even today. During the Christmas season, he forgot my birthday in early December. A loving and alert staff member took him aside and helped him make a birthday card. I love her for that tearful though joyful moment. Shortly after that, I gathered some of my favorite cards (birthday, Christmas, Mother's Day, Sweetest Day, "thinking of you") from our past twenty-six years that Don had personally selected for me from Hallmark's Mahogany collection, some with his own personal notations, and reread them. I love sharing my "cards collage" with others as I speak of my experience. The homemade card Don made is among them. What a joyful boost for me and a sweet remembrance for others who are seeking to make heaven out of the hell they are living!

That first year, even as Don's Alzheimer's progression increased, we found other joyful moments. You can too. Our dates included art exhibits with our Alzheimer's support group, walking in parking lots and adjacent neighborhoods, trips to the local barbershop (with Alzheimer's card in hand), or shopping at a local supermarket. Shopping for clothes at Kohl's—where Don's GQ wardrobe was replaced with standard khakis, sandals (sneakers with shoestrings no longer worked), and jeans—dining, of course, at KFC, and eating ice cream at a Brewster's outdoor patio were also among our dating times. When dining in other restaurants, Don selected the same menu item as me and suggested I handle the credit card payment. Occasionally, some of his trusted church friends would take him out as well. I made several vision boards for my own encouragement and focus. Here's two of them:

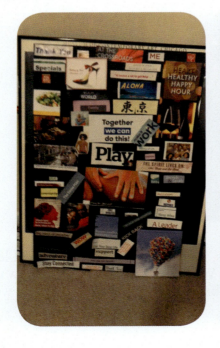

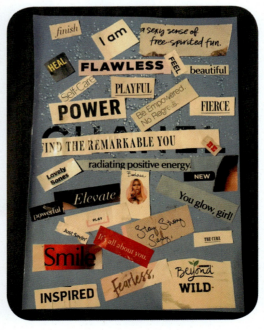

There were also intense times. Sometimes, walking on eggshells, I saw and heard things in this facility that were less than satisfactory. I chose to remember more with love than with pain. For example, Don began a "toilet protocol" about a year into his stay. His accidents were becoming more frequent, and staffers sought him out every two hours for a bathroom break. One particular staff member didn't stay on schedule but handled a difficult situation in good fashion. When she described what happened, I chuckled, joyful that she was involved and not me.

Don's bath time was another not-so-happy experience. Typically, Don took his showers at night, as I indicated in his "life snapshot" document. However, at the facility, staff awakened him early, 6:00 a.m., for baths. He fought, not wanting to be bothered. Now be honest—would you want someone bothering you for a shower early in the morning? He swung but missed at the female staff member. He did better with her male counterpart. I discovered that paid staff often perform tasks at their convenience and not on your loved one's schedule. I let them know that. I get that they have others to manage and are often short-staffed, but I got a small victory in this case. Staff started assisting Don's bathing during late mornings or in the afternoon instead.

Don is my rock; he now looks lost and confused much of the time.

I was overjoyed to be relieved of his medicine management schedule. They got it right every time. Don's hallucinations, decreased alertness, restlessness at night, fidgeting, moving things around with no purpose (remember, purpose was one of Don's characteristics), and bending to pick up imaginary things off the floor or in the air were common occurrences during this stage. When they seemed to heighten for no reason, however, I (not the staff) suggested he might have a UTI. I immediately took him to the doctor, who confirmed that it was. Stay in tune with your loved ones. You know them better than anyone. I was angry and upset when I took the prescription to the facility staff and informed them of his UTI. Hypervigilance was my game; I'd been doing it for several years now. My discovery of his pesky foot fungus too was because though he could not speak coherently, Don would cross his legs, pull his socks off, and scratch his feet. When I noticed an unusual smell (Don never had smelly feet!) and took a closer look, the tops of his feet were red and scaly with blackened soles. A doctor's visit confirmed my suspicions. Sometimes the facility reminded me of a petri dish, but Don was seldom sick. One other thing that perturbed me though—his glasses were frequently missing. After a not-so-nice encounter with the director, who insisted Don did have his glasses (in fact, they were not his), I eventually learned to get over it.

It was the UTI and foot fungus that drove me during the latter half of Don's second year of residency to request palliative hospice care for Don. Palliative hospice provides comfort, dignity, and more constant attention. *More* constant attention. Yes! Though the VA doctor admitted that Don was more confused and that the disease was progressing, he also said it was too early and did not advise hospice palliative care.

Instead, he said, "He'll live a long time."

My advice? Get a second opinion. Don's PCP (and also mine) approved the request. I was convinced that this move was appropriate as I recognized that another pair of eyes on Don would be helpful.

Hospice offers care, comfort, and dignity during the end of life. It is a great benefit, and I recommend it wholeheartedly. I was comforted knowing that more eyes would be on Don. Lord knows that I needed more monitoring to minimize and prevent falls that would exacerbate his brain bleeds. Although initially overwhelming, hospice was right on time. It was also around this time that Don began running into walls and windows and leaning to one side while walking. I thought he'd had a stroke. It was, in fact, accelerating Alzheimer's. His appetite remained good; I still often stayed and dined with him.

Activity directors in these facilities are worth their weight in gold. They do an amazing job celebrating birthdays and holidays. On weekends, I took Don's saxophone (remember, do not leave expensive items in these facilities) when I visited. He played solos, or when other residents sang, he picked up the tune on his horn. When Don played, his whole countenance changed. He went to another zone, somewhere that was happy, smooth, and pleasant. He would pat his feet and move his head. Music and dementia patients seem to go hand in hand. He also really enjoyed chewing gum with his mouth open; it seemed to relieve some of his stress and anxiety. He liked the minty kind best.

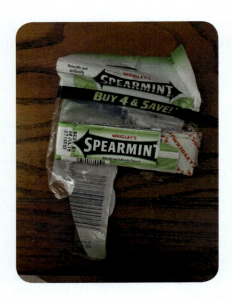

Most often, onsite support groups are part of the family benefits of long term care. I attended most of them. As his falls were increasing, Don slept in a high–low hospital bed with a scoop mattress, better known as a fall mattress. Two management staff members shared that Don was having difficulty sitting and holding his head up. He was frequently eating crazy food combinations with his hands (I remembered a similar incident from my previous book, *Mashed Potatoes in My Salad*). I was thankful he was still eating at all and getting some nourishment into his body. That was all that mattered—better than the time soon to come, when he would not eat at all.

> *And let us not be weary in well doing, for in due season, we shall reap, if we faint not.*
> — Galatians 6:9

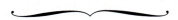

Other lessons I learned during this extremely difficult time were the following:

- Visit your loved ones in care facilities often and at irregular times.
- Become a vocal yet friendly advocate for your loved one.
- Maintain a good yet professional relationship with the facility staff.
- Always be kinder than you feel.
- Make the most of your time with your loved one.

- Daughter Nicole remarked once, "When Don's engaged, he is engaging." She was so right. During times of Don's incoherent rambling speech, I would often call his name and say, "That is it." "I think so." "It was good, babe." "Wouldn't that be nice?" He would stop, turn, and smile.
- Create memories; then create some more.
- Begin a relationship with your local state ombudsman, the official appointed to investigate complaints against public authorities.
- Begin early in requesting benefits from the VA. Your experience can be infuriating and burdensome.
- Start making end-of-life preparations early.
- Trouble making decisions? Stressed, overwhelmed, or exhausted? Don't make any.
- Acceptance, compassion, patience, humor, appreciation, and the value of sleep are so critical in unnerving situations.
- Despite the distractions, be present, be patient, and be kind.
- Stay positive, uplifting, and encouraging.
- Stay vigilant. Look for signs of pain in your loved one: head held in hands, head bowed, or wincing.
- Consider fidget lap pads and weighted blankets, if appropriate, for your loved one.
- Drugs (Metformin, for example) may encourage the onset of dementia.
- Minor hearing loss contributes to dementia. Schedule a hearing test as part of your self-care.
- Always remember—it is better to have peace than to be right.

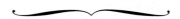

I do know that the way forward is to stay hopeful . . . but again, hope for what? I am still not sure. Perhaps just a better day tomorrow. As time continued to reveal what was coming ahead, I felt like the grip of grief was ongoing. I was not looking forward to what was next.

CHAPTER 7
Severe (Late) Stage Alzheimer's

For us, the severe (late) stage lasted about eighteen months. According to the Alzheimer's Association, severe stage symptoms of Alzheimer's include the following:

- Total care (comfort is the goal)
- Inability to communicate pain
- Little or no consciousness or awareness
- Sleeping most of the time
- Little meaningful communications with words
- Continued weight loss
- Unable to recognize family members
- Unable to recognize themselves in a mirror
- Falls
- Angry outbursts
- Vulnerability to infections

Don did recognize me and had no infections. His final Christmas, though, was fraught with mistakes and more falls. A recurring issue, constipation, along with inattention from several of the facility's staff, now required more intervention from me. Plus, his latest fall prompted a visit to the emergency room to assure Don did not have a concussion. By the time I got there, he was in a hospital bed, and they had already taken X-rays, indicating he had a subdural hematoma and blood on his brain (both old and fresh, from his numerous falls or having run into things). They also did not have his "do not resuscitate" (DNR) paperwork and suggested we move him to another hospital for surgery to have the blood drained. I said no, insisting that they read his DNR. He spent the night at the hospice facility. When we returned to the assisted living facility that afternoon, I proceeded to stay with him 24/7 until I could hire additional help.

For six weeks, I hired six sitters for around-the-clock coverage, in addition to his regular monthly expenses. I became an employer, of all things. The sitter service, though expensive, provided additional insight and confirmation into the unacceptable, less-than-satisfactory care from the facility's paid staff caregivers. One unexpected, joyful, and amazing moment I remember was when one of the overnight sitters I hired shared that Don prayed on two different occasions in the middle of the night. She mentioned that he was clear and concise in his petitions. From Don's margin notes in his well-used New International Version Holy Bible in 1 John 5:21, he wrote, "Be confident and bold with our prayers." What a joyful validation!

This situation came to a head as I searched for another alternative facility better equipped to handle Don's pressing needs and to stave off immediate financial concerns. In total, Don had long-term staff care, 24/7 companion/sitter service, and hospice palliative and regular care during his Alzheimer's journey.

On the recommendation of a previous staff member, I visited a memory care facility about thirty miles west of the current one. The care Don was receiving at the previous long-term facility no longer served his needs. Over the summer, his care was increasingly unsatisfactory. I was stressed as I watched so many assaults to his dignity. He sensed it. He seldom played his sax; nor did he finger the keys as he had done in the past. Don's medicines were adjusted to fight a persistent constipation problem. As moments of joy and sorrow are keys to our healing, I offered Don an apple, his favorite fruit. I was overjoyed as I watched Don go through his normal habit—rubbing the apple against his thigh, twisting it to remove the stem, and taking his first big juicy bite. That's how he ate and enjoyed apples.

Don seemed delighted about the move, though I don't recall talking about it in his presence. Still, when we were traveling there to visit, Don, sitting in the front passenger side of my car, with me in the backseat, mentioned to my daughter Erica, who was driving, that he was, in fact, ready to go and that it was time. To this day, I believe he *did* know.

My search for other resources to alleviate my financial condition was futile. We changed hospice services because the existing company was reluctant to visit him at the new facility. When the new hospice representative visited Don for her initial evaluation, she made these notes: he told her he wanted to go to church (his prayers weeks earlier indicated his faith in God prevailed and his desire to worship was alive). She also observed that Don was preoccupied; he was not in the moment but very active, intelligent, regimented, and perhaps a business owner (he had been). Further, she noted that his brain was looking for something to *do*; he needed to be engaged—he was a "young" eighty-year-old man with a youthful spirit about him. Oh, the joy that flooded my soul! Her final, frank notation was that at this stage, Don would continue to fall. For a short period, Don wore a specially designed helmet to prevent additional head trauma.

While he could still walk, we talked about his children, how he loved them and their love for him. I was thankful that Don was not wheelchair bound and that he did not suffer skin breaks, broken bones, bed sores, seizures, infections, or pneumonia, even though he was bedridden his last three weeks of life. Rather quickly, he moved from a slower, unsteady gait to no gait at

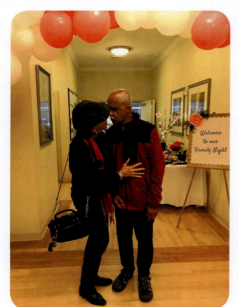

all. He had increased difficulty walking, eating, sleeping, and getting in and out of chairs. The loving, seemingly less rushed facility staff used chair-bound pillows to support his arms and legs. They used a particular chairlift to transport him. I am grateful that he did not have any stiffness in his joints or joint deformities. Don required intensive, around-the-clock care for all his needs now, including bathing, eating, dressing, bathroom breaks, and grooming. We went to our last Valentine's Day event before he was bedbound. I was slightly surprised when he leaned in and kissed me in this joyful moment.

At the new facility, he had visitors who would give me a break and walk with him around the building or offer communion. Other times, he and I spent time outside in the sunshine. I rubbed his hair and used gentle, reassuring touches on his arms, face, and legs. We looked at old photos in his well-worn books, though he was not as sure of their faces as he had been. We talked about good times. I read from his devotional books.

He seemed to listen. I played soft music as well, including his classical favorites like Bach and Handel and gospel songs like Brooklyn Tabernacle Choir and jazz tunes. Though his utterances lessened, I could tell he enjoyed our time. He was sleeping more during the daytime. It was during those times that I penned this short poem:

Keep it quiet.
Keep it calm.
Hold his hand.
Be his balm.

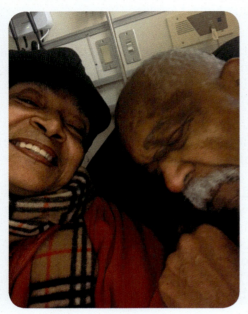

Decisions were already made during the diagnosis stage about life-sustaining treatments for him as the disease ravaged on. I am thankful for his caretakers during this time, who also kept his teeth and mouth cleaned and monitored bruises from his falls and his wincing from the brain bleeds. Perhaps the most heartbreaking episode for a caregiver is when their loved one barely eats and cannot swallow, choking on what they do eat. Don backed off eating noticeably and consistently near the end, about three weeks before his death. Before that, he had some trembling and was eating less, most often finger foods and sandwiches. We coaxed some fluids into him. Sometimes he only wanted a can of nutritional supplement.

However, the core of him remained. He purposely held hands with another resident, helping her walk down the hallway in his last days. Three weeks prior to his transition, Don lay in my arms on his bed and began to snore. I could not remember when I had last heard him snore. The restlessness and inability to relax had long prevented snoring. It was music to my soul! He looked so peaceful. His calm countenance was refreshing. I was not afraid. While the staff measured his intake and informed me regularly, I remembered this passage from my youth, knowing that we are not placed on this earth to stay:

> *Yea, though I walk through the valley of the shadow of death,*
> *I will fear no evil, for thou art with me.*
>
> — Psalms 23:4

I reflected on "the valley of the *shadow* of death." Shadows don't linger; they move on. Don looked peaceful. He looked so handsome. There was no strain, worry, or pain on his face this day. He smiled and appeared to be all right. Most days were not chaotic as plenty of people stopped in to make sure Don was comfortable. I was pleased. I thought of our life together, our wedding vows.

"Don, you loved me until death parted us," I said softly.

Someone else wrote this very appropriate four-liner:

I was supposed to spend the rest of my life with you,
And then I realized that you spent the rest of your life with me.
I smile because I know that you loved me 'til the day you went away
And will keep loving me 'til the day we are together again.

Here's my contribution to that sentiment:

Even so, my mind still talks to you,
And my heart still looks all over for you.
Because of you, I knew love,
But my soul confidently screams, "It is well!"
And knows you are at peace,
And for that, I am eternally grateful!

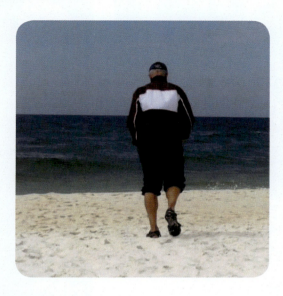

This ambiguous loss—bit by bit, slowly but surely—has been ongoing over the last eight years. I realized long ago Don would never return to his "Bub . . . bub . . . bub . . . bub . . . bub . . ." state of mind, that this loss of Don had already begun even before that utterance. My grief and my joy are connected by those joyful moments in between. Was this a death with dignity? Absolutely not, but I did my best to honor Don's request to "make sure I'm taken care of." Surely, he was in the grips of God's grace. These joyful moments will keep me forever.

I thank my God for every remembrance of you.

— Philippians 1:3

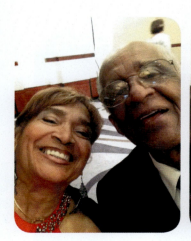 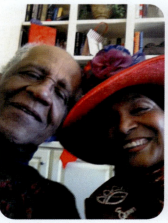 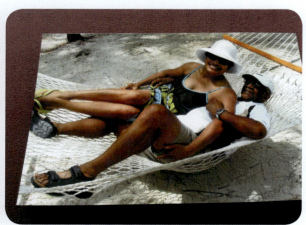

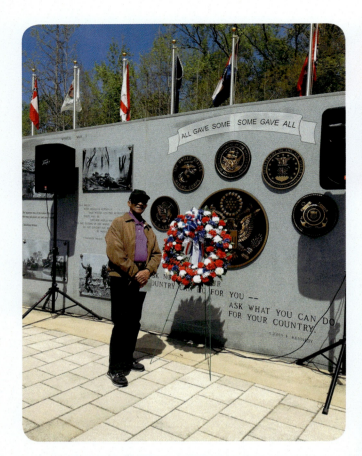

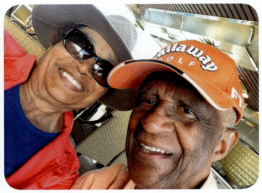

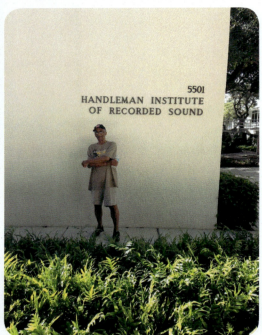

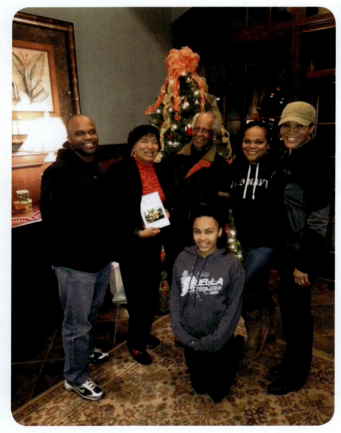

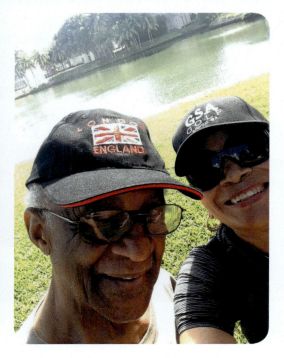

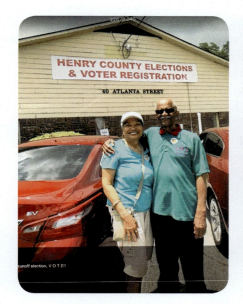

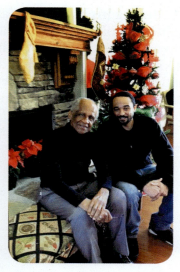

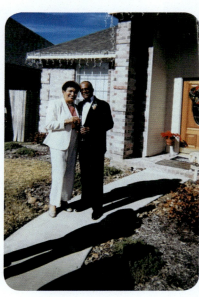

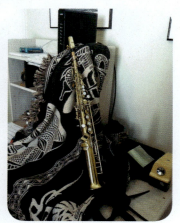

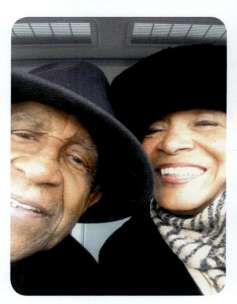

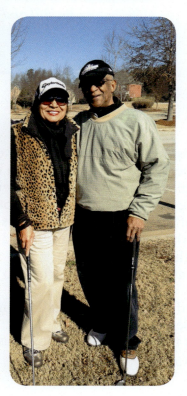

Of particular note during his last three days was when it appeared Don was unable to initiate engagement, daughter Nicole and her husband, Del, visited and brought two grandchildren, Kira and Nicholas, who were weeks away from high school graduation. When my son-in-law reached for Don's hand, Don grabbed his hand and held on. He interacted, smiled, and shifted with the grands as they chatted and posed for pictures. We all laughed and had a good time. I was reminded of Nicole's wise earlier observation: "When Don's engaged, he is engaging." Indeed, he was. I am thankful for that last joyful moment.

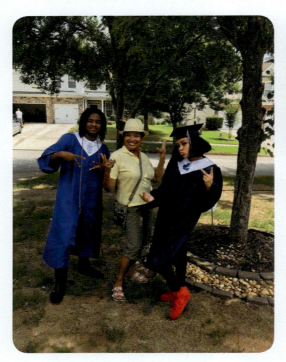 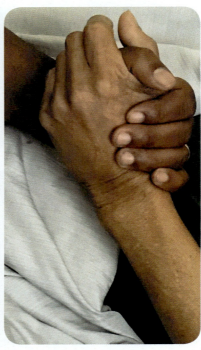

Be still and know that I am God.

— Psalms 46:10

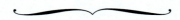

Other lessons of this season:

- When hospice service is refused by one member of your medical team, be persistent and try another. The right hospice team is invaluable.
- Our hospice team was the best. Their support group gave me comfort, joy, and strength, letting me know I was not on this road alone.
- Speak softly in your loved one's ears.
- Remove those who bring negative, draining energy to your space.
- Play soothing music often.
- Know that you did your very best to see your loved one through this journey. Have peace. It's time.
- Keep reading those devotionals or any favorites to your loved one. Personalize them. Their hearing senses are still keen.
- Consider that your long goodbye has come to an end. Be thankful and grateful and share that with your loved one.

CHAPTER 8
Don's Transition

Well done, good and faithful servant! Enter into the joy of the Lord.
— Matthew 25:23

Within forty-eight hours of our last family visit, Don's last earthly day was a busy one of hustling staff surrounding us and lovingly attending to him, quieting his termination agitation as his body prepared itself for the transition. I noticed that his breath changed at least six times. He slept continuously while I slowly and surely lost what was left of him, knowing that death—no, *freedom*—was imminent. Don's heart stopped at 11:45 p.m. on Tuesday, May 7, 2019. He transitioned gracefully and peacefully as he slept.

To be absent from the body is to be present with the Lord.
— 2 Corinthians 5:6

It was my honor to witness his incredible grit and fight along this journey. Surely, Don rests in the grips of God's grace. God's amazing grace shows up often. In this moment, I took note that we inhale our first breath out of the womb to begin life and that we exhale our last breath to end life and to leave this world. Amen!

Blessed are the dead who die in the Lord . . .
— Revelations 14:13

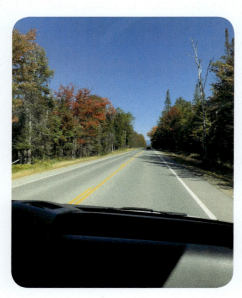

I was ready to get off this roller coaster ride, to rid myself of the twists and turns of Alzheimer's disease. With my heart and mind clear, I thanked God for this man of God, kissed Don's forehead, held his hand, tucked his covers, chatted with the hospice chaplain, waited until the funeral home representatives got there, and then drove home and went to bed, at peace that my man was at peace. This ambiguous loss is no longer ambiguous. Don has ultimate healing. It is well with his soul and with my soul. It was time to plan his celebration. Praise God!

I returned the next day and gathered Don's personal things. It was business as usual; the staff was preparing his room for the next occupant. I packed his clothes and placed them in my garage at home, where they stayed for over a month. The institutional odor lingered. I was not ready to be bothered. Hypersensitive? Yes, that's it—still.

Meanwhile, I exhaled deeply, for what was in front of me. I spent the week making the preparations for his service. I was overwhelmed, and handling the business of death was even more so—the discussions on a cause of death for the death certificate, notifying everyone, calling the minister, arranging the church details, selecting the music and participants, finding a funeral director, planning the celebration services, writing the service program and obituary, finding pictures, receiving the death certificate, canceling credit cards, switching names on accounts, closing bank accounts, calling the voter registrar's office, contacting social security and pension companies, responding to the outpouring of love and support, and then sorting through Don's personal items . . . so much to do!

Don's remains were cremated, and the uplifting celebration service was held a week later at our church. His beloved golf clubs and soprano saxophone were front and center as family and friends recalled and celebrated his life. Because Don was a veteran, his remains are buried at the Georgia National Cemetery in Canton, Georgia.

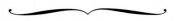

None of the previous deaths of loved ones close to me—dad, mom, aunties, uncles, siblings, in-laws—affected me like Don's death did. I loved my family members, though not in the intimate, closer-than-close, soul mate kind of way. Don was all of that and more for twenty-six years, so his death was very different. This experience was very much like a PTSD that I am slowly emerging from. The fog is finally lifting. Don and I reached the end of this long goodbye with mixed feelings. We actually seemed to enjoy the solitude knowing that the episodes were coming to a close, that his dignity was being restored, that the fighter had won the victory, that the preacher's words of "whole beyond again" finally made sense. For me, this never-before-experienced life event represented a new chapter in my life. Moving from soul mate to wife and then widow was weird. It was going to take time getting used to my life-altering shift. Don had a new body in a new home. As I reminisced while Don slept for hours before his calm and quiet transition, beautiful memories of the best husband I've ever had—I'd always said that—flooded my soul. Those joyful memories among the horrors of this disease are shared within these pages. Use them to recognize and find your own.

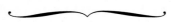

The lessons continue:

- Life's challenges force you to grow in ways you never imagined.
- Get up and go find your joy . . . Recharge.
- Get help; this life-changing event has many repercussions.
- Join a grief support group.
- The sun will shine again.

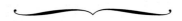

Finally—and with mixed feelings—I'm looking forward to what's next, to clawing my way back to me. A new chapter of my life is on the horizon. I do know that the way forward is to stay hopeful—always hope. Though the grip of this journey has eased, my grief journey yet awaits me. I'll do the work—slowly, gently, at my pace, extending to myself grace.

May the God of hope fill you with all joy and peace as you trust in Him . . .
— Romans 15:13

CHAPTER 9
Moving Forward

Without You

I never imagined living without you.
Then a red cardinal landed in the fairway and
looked in my eyes.
I stopped abruptly, smiled, and said,
"Get outta the way, Don, so I can hit this golf
ball!"
Fore! Ever in my life . . .
Always.

I never imagined living without you.
Another red cardinal, perched on the fence
next door,
Right in my line of sight
As I spoke of you on the phone
To my Alzheimer's support group.
You assured me of your ever presence
In my life—
Always.

I never imagined life without you—
A life minus Alzheimer's, yes.
My sleep is better, though I heard a "babe"
call out
Outside our bedroom door.
I've stopped taking the anti-anxiety pills.
I like the back to me I'm seeing—
Finally.

I never imagined life without you
As grandson and I shared your July 4 visit,
For him a favorite tune, "I'm in Love," at
hole #18,
For me a persistent, never-before light flicker
on your side of the closet.
Your presence is intense, your aura over all
of us—
Always.

I never imagined living without you,
But here I am, a woman emerging
From eight devastating (horrific) years of
Alzheimer's caregiving,
Lovingly giving you the best that I had to give,
An emotional, physical, mental, financial war
of an uphill—no, roller coaster—ride,
After doing my best to move heaven and earth
at my own expense to care for you,
My beloved.
All is well.

Whose patience had reached its limits, whose
resilient "snap back" tendencies were tested,
Who saw and did things she should not have
seen and did for her spouse,
Who made life-and-death decisions that no
one should have to make,
With battle scars—seen and unseen—that
have yet to be healed
Whose life gradually changed into a living
nightmare and who managed to hold it
together—most of the time.

I never imagined living without you,
Fighting the battle of a lifetime.
What a journey, a wonderful life fading before
my very eyes!
We had whatever we wanted, together and
separately.
Your transition freed both of us, gave peace to
both of us. We fought a losing battle that
Turned out to be a winning victory . . . your
heavenly home.
The shadow of death has passed.
You were ready to go; your body was worn and
tattered.
You rest, and I rest, for "it is well with my soul."
A new beginning awaits, and you are right here
beside me.
You are at peace; you are free!
It's a new beginning, a new chapter
For me.

Weeping may endure for a night, but joy comes in the morning.

— Psalms 30:5

My journey back to me is in fits and starts. I am not lazy, unmotivated, or stuck after years of living my life as the sole caregiver to Don. Rather, I am totally exhausted. Get that. The goal for me is to honor Don by living my best life *better*. I am getting there. This journey has emptied me; the pain and trauma of widowhood is overwhelming. There's no getting over it or moving on, just moving forward and savoring the joyful moments. This death of my husband from such a devastating terminal illness has literally changed my life. Every single thing in my world going forward is different—how and what I eat, whether to cook, sell the kitchen (which I've threatened to do), dine out, make or develop new connections, accept that old friends are different or nonexistent, watch TV, adjust to changed family dynamics, keep new friends, and recover my scattered finances. My self-worth, self-esteem, confidence, rhythms, thoughts, hobbies, interests, sense of security, sense of humor, sense of womanhood, sense of purpose, and life-altering experience converging to the now are different. *Different*. Yes, so very different.

For me, the grief stage lasts however long it lasts. I've experienced the classic grief characteristics backward, forward, upside down, and right-side up: denial, anger, bargaining, depression, and acceptance. They often take on various forms. Sometimes it feels like rocks inhabit my being; other times, it feels like I'm sinking in an ocean. It's been over a year since my beloved Don transitioned. That year went slow and fast as each milestone—Mother's Day (which was a week after Don's death), Independence Day, Labor Day, Don's eight-first birthday in October, Thanksgiving, Christmas, New Year's, Easter, and then his transition date of May 7 and his celebration service on May 17—came and went.

In that first year, I made no major decisions, putting everything on hold. I wanted to sleep, sleep, and sleep some more. Meanwhile, life was waiting.

One morning I woke up, showered, put on clothes and lipstick, combed my hair, looked at my reflection in the mirror, and said, "I am pleased."

I survived to share the journey, on my time, at my convenience, in any format I choose.

Aloud, I said to no one in particular, "What's up for today, girlie?"

I'm free to travel, roam, golf, dine, wine, nap, visit—anything of my choosing, even at the last minute. I liked that. New beginnings and new possibilities exist. I announced plans to sell my kitchen (no takers yet!). My new role of taking care of me is a priority. I mentally confirmed my new self-care support team: godly women, financial planners, practical bosom buddies, encouragers, spiritual partners, got-my-back grief support groups, and the Alzheimer's spouse group. I know I don't have to go forth alone. I won't. For that, I am grateful.

That fall, I began a recovery, restoration, and healing travel itinerary, spending time in Tennessee, and then witnessed the changing seasons of foliage colors straight out of the Crayola crayon box in the New England states (New Hampshire, Vermont, and Maine). After that, I headed to Chicago and golfed in the nearby states of Wisconsin, Indiana, and Iowa. Utah was next for a wholistic retreat and then south to Houston, Texas, and finally the beaches in Florida to calm my battered being. I was preparing an encore session, perhaps even international getaways. Then *bam!* The year 2020 began with rumblings of a worldwide coronavirus, commonly known as COVID-19. I wasn't ready. I still needed family, hugs, kisses, connections, outings, and lunches. I needed to touch and be touched. I was so touch deprived.

Instead, isolation, social distancing, masks, mask acne, limited or no travel, opened windows, and a quarantine routine interrupted my getting-back-to-me journey. I could not touch a hand, engage in a kiss or a face-to-face touch, lay a head on a shoulder or an arm around a neck—nada! My psyche was and is extremely affected. With masks, there is no need for even lipstick, my favorite makeup booster. Recently, in a virtual yoga class, we hugged ourselves—stretched our shoulders—and I cried! Left arm over right, right arm over left, I cried both times—touch deprived, indeed. COVID-19 is now prolonging my grief. I am still beyond distraught; I needed more time to get back to me.

If there is an upside to COVID-19, one is that quarantining has provided time for some much-needed home maintenance. Outdoor painting, staining, garage repairs, power washing, lawn care, rock painting, and patio decorating keep me busy. Over time, I've accumulated many travel-size toiletries that I am now using daily as I have no plans to fly anytime soon. I'm learning more about my iPad, reading piles of books, going through bottles of nail polish as I give myself manicures and pedicures, organizing and cleaning my golf shoes and my bedroom closet, and listening to my music collection on albums, CDs, and cassette tapes. Of course, I am writing. This book was birthed, finally. Surprisingly—blessedly—I never stopped golfing; it is naturally a socially distant sport.

How else has Don's transition affected me? From a practical standpoint, I still consider how to get to Don's long-term facility site from wherever I am when I am out and about, as if I were still going to visit him every day. On a trip to a local mall, I encountered a mannequin dressed in navy corduroy pants and had a meltdown; Don loved his corduroy pants. My first tuna sandwich from Subway was over a year after Don's transition, and I couldn't eat it all. Still, my cell phone is no longer easily accessible for emergency calls, especially on the golf course; it is intentionally hidden deep in my pocket. Unsettling societal problems of unwarranted killings, protests, marches, police issues, and political unrest have added to my stress levels. Surely, I am a different person, a better person, one who is more grateful, more present, more aware of how precious life is. Young people call it "woke."

I don't sweat the small stuff, and it's all small stuff. I've come to realize that I need to be with people still going through or beginning this journey. Therefore, I continue reaching out to the Alzheimer's and caregiver community to encourage and share my story, hoping someone will get a nugget of joy. I readily consult with and speak one-on-one with others who are going through this traumatic experience. I continue being involved in Facebook private groups where I can learn from others, offer insights, and encourage them. I still attend many conferences, workshops, and other Alzheimer's-related venues that provide valuable information and insights into this destructive disease. I am forever hopeful for a cure, a different protocol, a scientific breakthrough and will likely continue supporting these events indefinitely. There is still a need for the voice of the unpaid, loving caregiver. The people I've met along the way are dedicated, informed, and awesome, and many are lifelong friends.

Although I am resilient and adaptive, I no longer tolerate people who have no interest in my well-being or who have hidden agendas. Most people who say, "I know what you are going through" do not know what I am going through. I avoid them.

I engage in humor and laughter at every chance. Funnyman Steve Harvey is often my comedic break. I also love romantic comedies and old comedy shows like *The Carol Burnett Show* and *I Love Lucy* and the movies *It's Complicated* and *As Good As It Gets*.

I remain active; golf, Zumba, yoga, gym classes, and travel keep me busy (pre–COVID-19). Most days, I leave my home at noon and stay out and about until 3:00 p.m. It's a sanity check. Under different circumstances, Martin Luther King Jr. said something that perfectly fits my situation:

If you can't fly, then run.
If you can't run, then walk.
If you can't walk, then crawl.
But whatever you do, you have to keep moving forward.

I move forward at my pace. I am still removing Don's voice mail to me from my cell phone. I still look at videos of him dancing. I'll likely keep those. I'm still boosting my joy.

Though I doubt I'll ever marry again, I am open to dating. Here's my COVID-19 spin on getting together:

Dating COVID-19 Style

At a season in life when one finds that they are single—
Whether deliberate, divorced, career focused—one still desires to mingle.
Surely, for those hesitantly ushering in widowhood,
Dating becomes a murky situation, frequently misunderstood.

With all the usual stuff—why, when, who, where, and how—
It's even more difficult, considering the here and now,
For COVID-19 causes us to reconsider what a date looks like,
A vivid imagination, what exactly makes the journey right.

No dining, no drinks, no theater or sporting events,
Pressed to get to know one another without these accoutrements—
Whether to go forward or stay put is the thoughtful tone,
Out-of-the-box thinking or staying home alone.

After ninety-plus days of coronavirus affliction,
Singlehood often is the least of the friction.
No touchy, no kissy, no hugs, and social distance—
Six feet apart is your all-consuming Christian witness.

Yes, God indeed has a strange sense of humor.
How 'bout a one-on-one backyard in a place called outdoors,
Chef Longhorn's or Marco's pizza for dinner a la carte,
Bug spray, sunscreen, wine service from the local mart?

Thankful that springtime is in the air,
More options to think of besides the usual fare.
BYOE means bring your own everything,
To feel at home, relax, listen to the birds sing.

One final thought: don't forget your seeing glasses.
Add those masks, cover-ups—any style passes,
For this bold pandemic is unlike any other—
Air hugs, waves, Wakanda stances, lest you smother.

Walk to the car, bid farewell, say, "I had a good time."
Then decide where you're going next—your place or mine!
Sweet dreams.

I get an annual memory screening and a hearing screening since mild hearing loss contributes to dementia. You should too.

While I tried coping with my graying hair, to be honest, I just cannot. So I continue to indulge in my hair-coloring adventures, often some shade of red or brown. I did purchase two gray wigs; however, I don't like them. Need one? You can have them both. I am comforted by the words of St. John Chrysostom: "Those whom we love and lose are no longer where they were before. They are now wherever we are." Don visits me often. He never saw me with gray hair. I am blessed.

Finally, a good friend noted six months after Don's passing, "You look good. How are you?"

Thanking her, I replied, "I'm putting one foot in front of the other, moment by moment. Forward is my goal. Keep me lifted, for I feel your prayers."

To all of you reading this, please keep me lifted, and keep other caregivers lifted. I'm praying for you. Please know that you can do more than survive; you, too, can thrive. Peace!

Here are my final lessons.

- Don't deal with your grief alone. Find the right support group, including your hospice team.
- Don't be afraid to lean into grief. Do the work as grief runs deep, like a stain.
- Hold space for others who have your well-being in mind.
- Actively work on taking back your joy, whatever that looks like.
- Recognize false guilt. Eliminate words like *should*, *enough*, and *just*. Let it go.
- Maintain a sense of connection.
- Memories are forever, not just for now or for the moment. Collect them while you can.

EPILOGUE

The global COVID-19 pandemic arrived in the United States in January 2020. This virus created, among other things, a greater risk for social isolation, loneliness, depression, and dementia. As we are mainly social creatures and community minded, these harmful effects can attack healthy bodies. Under Alzheimer's caregiving, we already often feel alone and deserted by others. Signs like the lack of or too much sleep, gaining or losing weight, feeling tired often, losing interest in activities you normally would participate in, feeling worried or sad, and having body aches are magnified under COVID-19 restrictions, adding another layer of complexity. Yet, the world has slowed, and we are called to adapt.

Under the best circumstances, caregiving is both challenging and rewarding. The pandemic has created enormous, magnified disruptions and hardships that caregivers must manage for themselves and for their loved ones. These are unprecedented times. Services such as adult day care and respite care options have closed their doors or dwindled. Visits to doctors have switched to phone calls and virtual appearances. As caregivers, it is important that we keep ourselves and our loved ones calm and comfortable. COVID-19 guidelines—including wearing masks, keeping appropriate distances, staying out of crowds, and washing your hands—go against creating a soothing environment.

Quarantines have placed restrictions on our visits to loved ones in long-term care facilities and to loved ones receiving necessary care in their homes. Sickness and death have taken their toll on all of us. Death even looks different. Though steadfast in commitment to service, our hands are tied during this pandemic. Virtual technologies replace many hands-on, high-touch moments that are critical to us managing our loved ones. Still, we must keep well by moving, exercising, and creating safe spaces. Many of the safeguards currently in place are difficult under normal circumstances: washing hands for twenty seconds, using sanitizer, disinfecting high-touch areas, keeping hands away from your face, practicing social distancing, limiting interactions with others, restricting hugs and kisses, and fists bumps instead of handshaking or handholding. These measures are counter to crucial connections with loved ones who have serious, chronic illnesses or, in this instance, Alzheimer's.

We have been living under COVID-19 for nearly a year, and the effects of staying in touch with friends and family and your loved ones are challenging. The things you used to do to keep your loved ones engaged can no longer be done in the same way. Your visitation times have been altered. Your time for respite or to run errands has been curtailed. What little remains of your health and wellness under caregiving has taken a hit, and your loved ones suffer too.

Be encouraged. Stay flexible and open-minded. Many of the social engagement activities like painting, singing, playing an instrument, walking, scavenger hunts, and folding (and refolding) laundry can be done using FaceTime or through one of the social networking media platforms. Working collaboratively with your care team makes a huge difference. Where there's a will, there's a way. For example, if you can take a drive to the nearest strip mall and walk the outer perimeters, leave your environment daily (if you can), if only to drive and park and observe. If you've a lakefront, spend time there. Get out as much as possible. Regularly place calls to others in your network; don't wait for them to call you. Reach out. Send your loved ones a small gift. Better yet, deliver it within sight of your loved one. When people come together to help one another, progress is made, and our loved ones benefit. You can do this.

As we learn to maneuver this conundrum with kindness to ourselves and loved ones (even when we don't feel like it), don't forget to deeply breathe, pray, meditate, rest, laugh, stay social, refer to this book, and emphasize the positive. Share strategies. Remember that while you are having fun, you are also making joyful memories that will last a lifetime. The advice of Don's speech therapist still holds true: "Focus on the things that you can do, not what you cannot do." Seek grace for your place. You can do this. Remain happy and joyful. This, too, will pass.

RECOMMENDED REFERENCES AND RESOURCES

Alzheimer's Association (ALZ.org)
Help Me Help Momma
Home Instead Senior Care
Us Against Alzheimer's
Blog-writing websites
American Association of Retired People (AARP.org/caregiving)
Alzheimer's Foundation of America
Veteran's Administration
African American Network Against Alzheimer's
Alzlive.com
AlzheimersDisease.net
Emory Goizueta Alzheimer's Disease Research Center
CaraVita Home Care (in-home care services)
Support groups (widows/widowers, spouse, family members)
Podcasts: Lon Keiffer's thecaregiverpodcast.com (11/2019; search for Eunice Sykes)
Teepa Snow
Caregiving Institute at the Carter Center
National Family Caregiver Support Program
Facebook private groups
Area Agency on Aging
Hospice
State Ombudsman Contact
November is National Alzheimer's Disease Awareness Month, and June 21 is "the Longest Day" for Alzheimer's celebrations (annual).

Books:

The 36-Hour Day, Fifth Edition (Dr. Peter V. Rabins and Nancy L Mace)
Caring for a Spouse with Dementia (Kathy Bowen)
Hope for the Caregiver (Peter Rosenberger)
The End of Alzheimer's (Dr. Dale Bresden)
Mashed Potatoes in My Salad: An Alzheimer's Caregiver Memoir (Eunice L. Sykes)

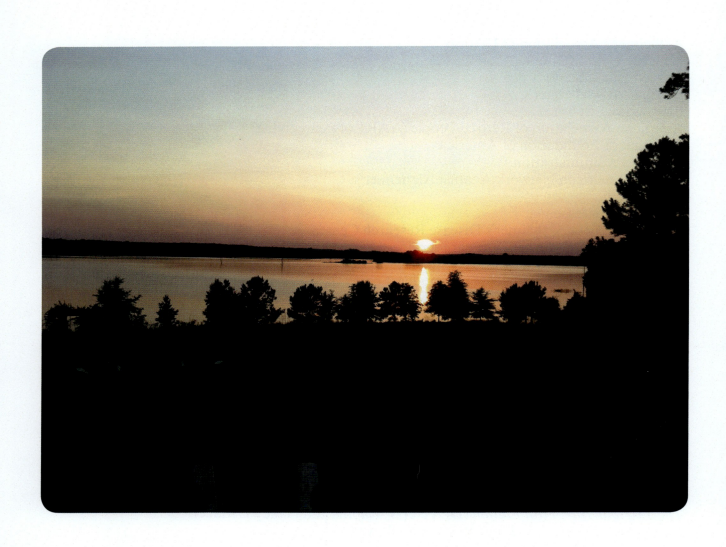